SUPERVISION AND ITS VICISSITUDES

The EFPP Clinical Monograph Series

Editor-in-Chief: *John Tsiantis*

Associate Editors: *Brian Martindale* (Adult Section)
Didier Houzel (Child & Adolescent Section)
Alessandro Bruni (Group Section)

OTHER MONOGRAPHS IN THE SERIES

Countertransference in Psychoanalytic Psychotherapy with Children and Adolescents

Supervision and Its Vicissitudes

edited by

Brian Martindale

SENIOR EDITOR

Margareta Mörner

María Eugenia Cid Rodríguez

Jean-Pierre Vidit

Foreword by

Robert S. Wallerstein

Routledge
Taylor & Francis Group
LONDON AND NEW YORK

for

The European Federation
for Psychoanalytic Psychotherapy
in the Public Health Services

First published 1997 by Karnac Books Ltd.

2 Park Square, Milton Park, Abingdon, Oxfordshire OX14 4RN
52 Vanderbilt Avenue, New York, NY 10017

Routledge is an imprint of the Taylor & Francis Group, an informa business

First issued in hardback 2019

British Library Cataloguing in Publication Data
Supervision and its vicissitudes
1. Psychoanalysis
I. Martindale, Brian
150.1'95
A C.I.P. for this book is available from the British Library

ISBN: 978-1-85575-161-3 (pbk)
ISBN: 978-0-367-32716-3 (hbk)

Edited, designed, and produced by Communication Crafts

ACKNOWLEDGEMENTS

I would like to thank a number of people who have been important in the bringing of this monograph to completion. Especial thanks must be reserved for all the chapter authors, who have been exceptionally industrious and helpful throughout. The following translators are gratefully acknowledged: Vivienne Sarobe and Françoise Soetens for chapter one, Françoise Soetens for chapter three, Christine Ernsting for chapter four, Judith C. Leemann for chapter five, and Sheila Smith for chapter nine. Particular thanks are also due to Philippa Martindale, who spent many hours working on improvements to the text and the reference section, and to Eric King for the final copyediting.

I would also like to acknowledge the important contributions of the editorial team of Margareta Mörner (Sweden), María Eugenia Cid Rodríguez (Spain), and Jean-Pierre Vidit (France).

I am also most grateful for all the support and advice I have received from both John Tsiantis, the editor-in-chief of the EFPP Clinical Monograph Series, and Cesare Sacerdoti of Karnac Books.

The EFPP wishes to express its sincere gratitude to the Association of Psychoanalytic Psychotherapy (British National Health Service) and Riksforeningen Psykoterapi Centrum (Sweden) for their generous financial contributions towards the costs of production of this monograph.

Brian Martindale
London, April 1997

ABOUT THE AUTHORS

KURT GORDAN, PSW, PhD, is an assistant Professor of Psychology and a Psychotherapist in private practice. He was Director of the Erica Foundation in Stockholm, 1970–1988. He trains senior psychologists, psychiatrists, and social workers in psychotherapy and supervision. He is a Consultant and Supervisor to public institutions for health care, theatre, etc. He is the author of books about antisocial adolescents, psychotherapy supervision, and professional "encounters".

LEÓN GRINBERG, MD, is a Training and Supervising Psychoanalyst for the Madrid Psychoanalytic Association and also a Member of the Buenos Aires Psychoanalytic Association. He is a former Vice-President of the International Psychoanalytic Association and President of the Argentine Psychoanalytic Association. He has been a Professor at several institutions. He has lectured in numerous countries and is the author of many books which have been translated widely.

ROBERT LANGS, MD, is Visiting Professor of Psychiatry at the Mt. Sinai School of Medicine in New York City and Visiting Clinical

Researcher at the Nathan S. Kline Institute for Psychiatric Research in Orangeburg, New York, and Honoured Visiting Professor at Regent's College School of Psychotherapy and Counselling, London. He is a Member of the American Psychoanalytic Association. He lectures and teaches in many countries and is the author of many books and papers in the fields of psychotherapy and psychoanalysis.

DOROTHY LLOYD-OWEN is a Psychoanalytic Psychotherapist and an Associate Member of the British Association of Psychotherapy, where she is on the Training Committee. She trained and worked previously as a Senior Probation Officer. She works at the Portman Clinic in London and in private practice.

BRIAN MARTINDALE, MRCP, MRCPSYCH, is a Consultant Psychiatrist in Psychotherapy at Parkside Clinic and St Charles Hospital, London. He trained at the Maudsley and Cassel Hospitals and is an Associate Member of the British Psychoanalytic Society. He was the founding member and Past Chairman of the European Federation of Psychoanalytic Psychotherapy and is on the executive board of the International Society for the Psychological Treatments of Schizophrenia and other psychoses. He has published in a number of areas including psychoanalytic psychotherapy with the elderly.

MONTSERRAT MARTÍNEZ DEL POZO, PhD, is a Psychologist and a Child, Adult, and Group Training Psychoanalytic Psychotherapist. She is President of both the Spanish Association of Psychoanalytic Psychotherapy and the Catalan Association of Psychotherapists and is a Spanish group section delegate to the EFPP. She is a staff member of the Clinical Psychology Service of the Fundación Puigvert, Hospital de la Santa Cruz and San Pablo, Universidad Autónoma de Barcelona, and a Professor and Supervisor at various institutions. She has published, with colleagues, a number of books on work with children, adults, and groups.

PETER-CHRISTIAN MIEST, LIC. PHIL, is a psychoanalyst and member of the Swiss Psychotherapy Association (SPV) as well as a supervisor in private practice in Basle, Switzerland.

VICTOR SEDLAK, PhD, researched into learning disabilities before training as a Clinical Psychologist in Leeds and as a Psychoanalytic Psychotherapist at the Tavistock Clinic. He is now a Member of the British Psychoanalytical Society and in recent years has moved back to the north of England, where he is interested in the development of psychoanalytic psychotherapy and psychoanalysis in that region. He has also been active over many years in Poland, promoting similar developments. He has published on topics such as assessment, dreams, countertransference, and work with psychotic patients.

ULRICH STREECK, MD, MA, is a Psychiatrist, Psychoanalyst, and Sociologist. He is Professor and Medical Director of the Tiefenbrunn Clinic and Hospital for Psychotherapy, Psychiatry, and Psychosomatic Medicine of Lower Saxony in Germany. He is Past President of the German psychoanalytic umbrella organization (the DGPT). He has conducted qualitative psychotherapy research on psychotherapeutic dialogues, group psychotherapy, and in-patient psychotherapy and is the editor of several books on clinical psychoanalysis and qualitative research.

IMRE SZECSÖDY, MD, PhD, is a Psychoanalyst and is President of the Swedish Psychoanalytic Society. He is Associate Professor at the Karolinska Institute, Stockholm. He was the director of the West Stockholm County Psychotherapy Training Unit. He has conducted extensive research into supervision and the learning process and has long experience of conducting the formal training of supervisors. He has published extensively.

ROBERT S. WALLERSTEIN, MD, is Emeritus Professor and former Chairman of the Department of Psychiatry, University of California San Francisco School of Medicine. He is a Training and Supervising Analyst at the San Francisco Psychoanalytic Institute and was President of the American Psychoanalytic Association (1971–1972) and President of the International Psychoanalytical Association (1985–1989).

CONTENTS

FOREWORD

Robert S. Wallerstein

It is by now a truism that though the supervisory process has increasingly emerged over recent decades as the central vehicle in the teaching of psychoanalysis and psychoanalytic psychotherapy, there is still a much-decried paucity of literature on its nature and its vicissitudes, and even less empirical research study of the supervision process, or specific training programmes equipping one with the requisite supervisory capacities. Originally, of course, psychoanalysis began with a tripartite model for psychoanalytic training, with the three major components—the personal analysis, the didactic seminars and conferences, and the conduct of psychoanalysis under supervision—at least conceptually of equivalent importance, and this model has, indeed, persisted almost unchallenged since its initiation by Max Eitingon with the founding of the first formal psychoanalytic training institute in Berlin in 1920. But it has also all along been acknowledged that, in practice, the three component arms have never been accorded equal status.

For a long time, many placed the personal analysis as the central element in the formation of the psychoanalyst. But over the most recent decades the psychoanalytic world has clearly moved towards an increasing consensus that the personal analysis of the psychoanalytic candidate should be, as far as is humanly possible, just that—an unfettered therapeutic activity, removed totally, again as far as is humanly possible, from pedagogical considerations and the educational progression. There is, indeed, ample literature on this issue. All this has, concomitantly, moved the supervision process to centre stage as the primary experiential vehicle in the educational formation of the psychoanalyst and, *pari passu*, of the psychoanalytic psychotherapist. And yet, as has been made clear in several of the chapters in this monograph, the relative sparseness of the literature devoted clinically and theoretically to supervision as a helping process—very distinct from, albeit related to, therapeutic processes on the one hand, and to formal school educational processes on the other—has remained unaltered. And beyond that, of course, there continues to be even less systematic study and formal research devoted to the supervisory process of the kind described here by Imre Szecsödy, or formal training programmes to educate clinicians into the skills and attributes of the supervisor of the kind described here by Kurt Gordan, both of whom are from Sweden.

In fact, Rudolf Ekstein introduced just such a programme of educating (by supervising) the supervisors, via individual consultation sessions and a supervision seminar, into The Menninger Foundation training programmes in the 1950s, which was the organizing nidus for our joint 1958 book, *The Teaching and Learning of Psychotherapy*. This programme, however, was never institutionalized or made the basis for the accreditation of supervisors, as it now has, seemingly so successfully, in Sweden. It is, rather, still the near-universal experience in clinical training programmes around the world that one becomes a supervisor and teacher with no special preparation or training for the role, but just by having demonstrated adequate competence as a clinician and therapist.

For these and many other reasons, this present monograph by the EFPP is indeed a very welcome and very substantial addition to the still all too scanty literature devoted to this centrally important topic of supervision. A main contribution of this monograph, as I see it—and one not developed elsewhere in the supervision literature as I know it—is in detailing and exemplifying, through cumulative instances, Ekstein's own original statement of credo about supervision: that it is a generic interpersonal (i.e. emotionally charged) helping and learning process, grounded theoretically perhaps in the psychoanalytic understanding of mental functioning, but applicable across an entire spectrum of interpersonal helping situations, from those that demand the most extensive and technically complex training to those that require the very least.

The progression of chapters in this monograph distinctly exemplifies this thesis. The first chapter, by León Grinberg of Spain, is clearly drawn from and focused upon the problems and issues in the supervision of psychoanalytic candidates—those in the most intensive and rigorous training for the most ambitious reconstructive efforts directed towards maximal personality restructuring, and much beyond just the amelioration of behavioural and symptomatic distress. It is a training in which the supervisory teaching is built solidly upon both the personal analytic therapy of the student and the intensive several-year-long clinical and theoretical seminar sequence. However, the very next chapter, by Victor Sedlak of the United Kingdom, based on work in England away from the educational richness of London and in Poland, where psychodynamic therapy has so recently emerged from under the cloud of official Communist interdiction, extends the supervisory considerations—necessarily adapted, of course, to these differing circumstances—to the training of psychodynamically concerned and interested, but essentially untrained, therapists. And in doing this, Sedlak brings us back to one of the two major roots of our supervision experience and knowledge: the first, exemplified here in Grinberg's chapter, was traditionally in psychoanalysis, with the supervision built upon the prior personal therapy of the therapist; the other, and on which Sedlak builds, was in psychiatric social work, where from the start personal therapy was not expected or required—unless recommended on the basis of supervision that encountered insuperable personal, i.e. countertransference, problems in the supervisee—and where the burden of the learning process and the acquisition of skill as a caseworker and therapist rested on the supervision alone (albeit with concomitant didactic teaching). The concept was that the "professional self" could be fostered as a therapeutic instrument without associated explicit attention to the "personal self"—unless the two, as indicated above, were too neurotically intertwined. Sedlak has skilfully advanced this important tradition.

The third chapter, by Montserrat Martínez del Pozo of Spain, has extended this ramifying net still further, to the carrying on of the supervisory work, grounded in psychoanalytic conceptions, into the psychotherapeutic activities undertaken in the public sector; in the latter, the private two-person therapeutic dialogue in the psychoanalytic or individual psychotherapeutic consulting room operates within the frame of an impinging, and at times constraining, public authority and public institution to which both the therapist and the supervisor are accountable. In the fourth chapter, by Ulrich Streeck of Germany, the ramifications are extended still further, beyond the supervisions of individual therapy, whether in a private therapeutic dyad or within a public institution with public accountability, beyond that to the supervision of working teams and team settings within institutional frameworks, where the various team members can represent different disciplines and/or different roles and tasks in relation to the patients in treatment in that setting.

And in what logically, in my mind, is the fifth in this growing arc of ramifying supervision situations, described in chapter six by Dorothy Lloyd-Owen of the United Kingdom, the supervisory concern is focused on forensic or legal-system therapeutic activity, with often unwilling patients court-ordered into psychotherapeutic contact as part of, or alternative to, incarceration for antisocial and criminal activities. Last, then, in the logic of this progression, is the work reported by Peter-Christian Miest of Switzerland in chapter five, where those being supervised are not directly mental health professionals of any sort but, rather, simply those drawn as caretakers to terminally ill patients, mostly dying of AIDS, in a hospice setting, where indeed the caretakers are daily confronted with the most emotionally stirring interactions with their charges and all the most intense emotional reverberations upon themselves.

What is so beautifully exemplified in this entire sequence of chapters that I have depicted is how supervision, as a process conceptually grounded in the psychoanalytic understanding of mental functioning, is nonetheless a distinct process of its own, applicable generically to the whole range of helping situations—from the psychoanalyses carried out by the most intensively trained, to the nursing care and emotional support from caregivers in settings for the dying—although, of course, specifically adapted to the particular problems commonly activated in each of the settings described in these various chapters. To me, this demonstration of the universal applicability of an interpersonal supervisory helping process to such a spectrum of situations and contexts in which human emotional suffering is dealt with is the truly powerful—and inspiring—message of this monograph. It is the implicit underpinning of the whole; I wish only to make the point explicit.

For the rest, the monograph indeed has many other rewards for the reader. Space constraints permit me to allude only to some: the perspective on the parallel process as not only an important illumination of the issues in both the treatment that is supervised and the supervision of the treatment, but also as potentially a cover-up and a resistance to the uncovering of the transference, as indicated by Grinberg; the focus on the dialectic in supervision between "lack" and "conflict", as indicated by Szecsödy (restating in today's terms what Peyton Jacob inelegantly described, in the 1981 book I edited on supervision, *Becoming a Psychoanalyst,* as the back-and-forth between "dumb spots" and "blind spots"); the careful distinction between the countertransferences emanating primarily from the unresolved issues of the therapist (or the supervisor) and the projective counteridentifications of the therapist (or supervisor) but emanating primarily from the patient (or the supervisee), as described by Grinberg.

And finally one last point—in counterpart to the emphasis placed by Brian Martindale in his Introduction on an integrative perspective, on the commonalities that can indeed clearly be seen in this succession of windows on the supervisory process and its vicissitudes across such a variety of circumstances and contexts. I want, rather, to call attention, as I think I have through this whole Foreword, to the rich diversity and heterogeneity of perspectives on what supervision means and how it can best be conducted, ranging from the very rigorous and austere model presented by

Robert Langs of the United States, through the very traditional or "classical" model typified by Grinberg, to the much more (necessarily) relaxed models exemplified in several of the other chapters in this monograph. Overall it is, indeed, a feast for many appetites and many curiosities.

INTRODUCTION

Brian Martindale

Supervision of psychoanalytic therapy is increasingly recognized as requiring skills and knowledge somewhat distinct from that of being a competent psychotherapist. The literature on the theory and practice of supervision has expanded very considerably in recent decades, and in a few countries it is a requirement that supervisors have undergone specific trainings with proof of competence, in addition to trainings as psychoanalysts and psychoanalytic psychotherapists.

It may be of interest to seek valid explanations for the increasing maturity of the subject. Readers of this monograph will probably come to the conclusion that it is the growth both in sophisticated understanding of the different forms of countertransference and projective identification and of theories of "emotional learning" that has contributed most to the development of theory, practice, and training in supervision. Much of the supervision of work with more disturbed patients is likely to be beneficial if it focuses on unravelling projective and introjective identifications and the contribution that these forms of communication and defences of patients are making to the countertransferences of the staff.

Therefore, psychoanalytically based supervision is relevant not only to those in training to become individual psychoanalytic psychotherapists and for continuing post-qualification development. It also has considerable relevance and importance for those who are not specialist psychoanalytic psychotherapists but who encounter psychologically troubled persons in a wide range of settings. Like transference, countertransference is a ubiquitous phenomenon and mostly unconscious. If countertransference reactions are not able to be made conscious and reflected upon, there can be many forms of harmful enactments or verbal communications to patients or avoidance of emotional contact with them and their problems. The more disturbed the patient, the more likely are disturbing countertransferences and the more vulnerable is the patient to these reactions by staff. The additional problems and distress that staff themselves will suffer as a result of unconscious countertransference should not be minimized. Therefore, by identifying, containing, and understanding countertransference, skilled supervision can do much to improve the quality of psychological care given in mental health settings, whether or not various modalities of formal psychoanalytic psychotherapy are available.

This book is produced on behalf of the European Federation for Psychoanalytic Psychotherapy (EFPP), which is primarily concerned with the application of psychoanalytic ideas to work in the public sector. The book therefore contains a number of chapters that are specifically concerned with the type of supervision work with individuals, teams, and institutions that will often be in demand and useful in the public sector.

The first chapter is by León Grinberg of Spain, who gives a very comprehensive account of the definition, process, and vicissitudes of individual supervision in psychoanalytic psychotherapy and psychoanalysis. He focuses especially on transference and countertransference issues in the supervision itself. As do other chapter authors at many points in this book, Grinberg addresses the complex interface between the therapist's need for his personal therapy and the manifestation of his personal issues in his professional role, especially in his countertransference to the patient's material.* In

*For simplicity, in general discussions we have used the masculine pronoun.

what ways is it appropriate for the supervisor to engage with the supervisee and the latter's countertransference? Grinberg's own views are based on his clear theoretical differentiation between countertransference as usually currently defined and the very specific phenomena of projective counteridentification, which are states of mind in the therapist produced by the patient independent of the personal countertransference of the therapist. Grinberg carefully spells out these different categories of reaction in his text and gives his own guidelines to distinguish between what is appropriate for the supervisor to take up and what should remain only the province of the supervisee with his personal therapist.

The phenomenon of a parallel process between the therapeutic setting and the supervisory setting is one that has been found to be repeatedly observed and of usefulness in supervision. However, Grinberg illustrates that this phenomenon can be used by both supervisee and supervisor as a defensive cover for transference phenomena in the supervisor/supervisee relationship that in themselves may interfere with the supervision task. He goes on to give a considerable number of examples, firstly in supervisees, such as grandiose attitudes, greed that leads to swallowing rather than assimilation, contempt, rivalry, and envy. He then lists some problems of supervisors that can interfere with supervision, such as the consequences of professional isolation, as well as some remaining personality traits. Grinberg emphasizes the need for supervisors' capacity for concern in fostering the next generation (generativity).

Victor Sedlak, from the United Kingdom, focuses in the second chapter specifically on the supervision of therapists who have not had a full training. In many regions of Europe it is still very common for there to be very few well-trained psychoanalytic psychotherapists and psychoanalysts. Sedlak is surely correct in saying that it is important to be able to offer supervision to those professionals who are not fully trained but nevertheless are serious in their wishes to improve their work. It may be the most fruitful way of supporting local motivation to work towards proper training in psychoanalytic psychotherapy, and for this reason the chapter is of particular interest to those analysts and psychoanalytic psychotherapists concerned with regional development, such as those involved in developing the EFPP's networks.

Sedlak's chapter emphasizes the breakdown that occurs in psychoanalytic psychotherapy when the countertransference is not mastered. He gives a most interesting speculative interpretation of Freud's countertransference acting-out in his treatment of the Wolf Man, by the setting of a termination date (in the face of the endless repudiation of Freud's interpretative work). This occurred at a time before the complex pathology of destructive narcissism was fully understood. Sedlak then gives a very thorough account of a contemporary case from his supervisory practice in which the therapist started to act out his anxieties in the face of a patient's unconscious guilt, which had lead to a negative therapeutic reaction. The acting-out increased the patient's depression and despair. What is particularly important in this chapter is Sedlak's most instructive and open account of how he actually engaged with the therapist in thinking about the latter's countertransference difficulties and the consequences of that thinking for the success of subsequent therapeutic work. This sort of reporting is all too rare in the literature, yet surely this is the best way for good techniques to be debated and disseminated. In this particular case, it would be interesting to know whether León Grinberg would regard the therapist's responses in the situation reported as countertransference or as projective counteridentification.

In chapter three, Montserrat Martínez del Pozo from Spain describes supervision in institutional settings and focuses especially on a Klein/Bion framework. In the last twenty years, psychoanalysts in the Barcelona area have taken active steps to involve themselves in a teaching and supervision programme in the public sector, leading to substantial changes in the institutions that provide mental health care. Her chapter is based on the supervision now offered in such settings.

Through an example she emphasizes the constant fluctuations, in all parties involved, between more mature and more primitive states of mind when the material is difficult. Del Pozo uses an interesting term, "the learning position", translated from the French *alliance d'apprentissage,* a term believed to have been coined originally by Ludwig Haesler (Dispaux, 1994) to describe the supervisee's equivalent of the patient's therapeutic alliance in the supervisee/supervisor relationship. I think this will prove to be a most helpful phrase to describe the variable capacity of the supervisee to observe and struggle with his own responses and shifting states of mind to his patient's material and those evoked by the supervision.

Martínez del Pozo, through reference to ancient myths, brings "life-and-death issues", such as those when the supervisor also has the responsibility to support or hold back the supervisee at various stages in his passage through the training institution.

Chapter four is by Ulrich Streeck of Germany, who gives a particularly clear account of the potential spectrum of settings for skilled psychoanalytically based supervision in mental health settings. He also mentions the various attitudes and fears that may oppose these interventions. Streeck makes clear the importance of establishing the distinction between supervision for staff in their *professional relationships* and their work with patients, and *therapy for personal problems*. He also stresses the need for an accurate assessment of the nature and source of difficulties in an institutional setting before undertaking supervision to a particular group. In this way he highlights the fact that supervision is not an intervention that should always be offered whenever it is requested. By implication, he states that it is first necessary to assess whether the issues for which the individual or team are requesting help are likely to be best attended to by psychoanalytically based supervision or whether the major source of the difficulties is a manifestation of wider institutional or other problems. Having identified the location, it is then necessary to assess whether the problems are due to troubling unconscious emotional relationship factors, in which case psychoanalytically informed supervision may well be indicated, or to other sources such as those of a structural, organizational, or administrative nature.

The supervision methods that Michael Balint developed for engaging family doctors' interest in the psyche of their patients have spread widely to be used with many professional groups in the caring professions. The special group settings allow professionals to become more confident at noticing both their patients' unconscious communications and their own previously unconscious responses to these. The focus is on emotional factors as they occur in relationships between professional and patient, and the favourable consequence is a limited change or growth in the personality of the professional and therefore competence at addressing the psychological components of their practice.

The method is particularly suitable for offering skilled supervision to staff teams working in the public sector. The fifth chapter, by Peter-Christian Miest of Switzerland, is a clear example of a Balint-style group at work in a nursing home caring for people in advanced stages of AIDS. In this particular example, it is important to note how essential it was that careful thought went into the *setting* for supervision that the supervisor provided. Prior to the supervision, the multiple emotional factors that subsequently unfolded in the supervision had been denied and defended against by not creating a reflective space. However, the consequences of this denial had been serious, as manifested by the very high staff turnover from the unacknowledged emotional strains. As the supervision progressed, certain other spaces appeared that punctuated the busy times and allowed potential opportunities that parallel those rituals that society/cultures create to assist the mourning processes. This chapter offers a particularly useful illustration of the struggle in the supervision to identify the unconscious aggression and hatred of the staff towards their patients. On the surface, this was a deeply caring/loving staff group, and the uninformed observer might wonder why there should be a need to look behind this. Miest makes clear that the functioning of the institution was considerably handicapped by the highly disguised enactment of denied aggression, hatred, and also physical disgust, especially expressed by the high staff turnover, with its rejection of the institution.

Dorothy Lloyd-Owen of the United Kingdom highlights, in chapter six, the fascinating dynamics that emerge in primary forensic settings and sometimes lead to requests for supervision. She describes the typical forensic worker as often naively attempting to get the offender to engage with the superego of the worker! She portrays very clearly the complex institutional and societal pressures on the forensic service, especially the switching from magical expectations to ready denigration in the face of re-offending. Lloyd-Owen also highlights the changes in British Government attitudes, which have altered the whole atmosphere of the institutions connected with forensic care and reduced the chances of offenders being treated as whole persons and the consequent very painful issues that will therefore surface in supervision. Offering supervision to individuals in these circumstances might be seen to contradict some of the guidelines that Streeck lays down in his chapter. Lloyd-Owen's example of supervising social workers involved in a residential unit for abusing families gives striking evidence of the need to be able to help the worker to see the deleterious and harmful effects on their work of powerful projective identifications from the family if these remain unconscious. She ends by highlighting the problem posed for the workers as they acquire, through supervision, painful insights into the limits of the system within which they are working.

Imre Szecsödy of Sweden has spent many years studying and researching supervision. In chapter seven, he points out the biased emphasis in the literature and the many assumptions made in practice that have not been seriously questioned until recently. Examples include the assumption that an experienced and able psychotherapist will make a competent supervisor; the emphasis in the literature on how one teaches, rather than a focus on discovering how a supervisee learns; and the underestimation of the difficulty of the task of supervision. With respect to the learning process, Szecsödy's own research analysed transcripts of recorded supervisory sessions. He found that the different types of learning problem were not clearly delineated by supervisors, nor was the technique for attending to them. Problems based on lack of knowledge were not differentiated from problems based on the multiple conflicts of the trainee, such as those stemming from the training setting itself. He did find that learning was most likely to occur when the supervisor kept a stable focus on certain supervisory frames, especially the reconstruction of the interaction between supervisee and patient.

This last point brings us to Robert Langs' chapter (chapter eight) on the framework of supervision for psychoanalytic psychotherapy. Langs, who is from the United States, has written extensively on "communicative" psychotherapy. In this approach unconscious communications that stem from deviations and conformity with the framework in which psychotherapy takes place have a central focus of attention. Langs expounds his theoretical rationale and sets out the quite radical changes in supervisory style and technique that he believes should be followed as a consequence. It would seem, on the surface at least, that this is a very different theory and model of supervision from that espoused in other chapters. However, his treatise is based on the premise that contemporary psychoanalysis and psychoanalytic psychotherapy rarely focus on the frame and its deviations and that immediate deep unconscious significances are not decoded by therapists. Although there are many controversial points in the chapter, Langs will certainly provoke much thoughtfulness about contemporary supervision techniques.

The final chapter, by Kurt Gordan from Sweden, outlines a formal training in the supervision and teaching of (psychodynamic) psychotherapy. In Sweden it is now a requirement that supervisors and teachers of government-recognized psychotherapy trainings have themselves successfully completed training. The course that Gordan describes has already had twenty years of experience. It is clear that a lot of careful thought has gone into creating a teaching or learning framework whereby trainee supervisors and teachers can obtain accurate and immediate feedback on their own developing capacities to provide a setting in which emotional learning can take place. Gordan makes it clear that the training committee have to monitor carefully the temptation of the student group to focus on the contents of what they need to learn and teach at the expense of being exposed to crucial clarification as to how they were performing as teachers and supervisors. A first impression may lead one to believe that the approaches of Langs and Gordan are far apart, but I think that what the chapters in this monograph have in common is an interest in the factors in supervision that facilitate the therapist's emotional learning.

* * *

Previous publications on supervision have often stressed the poverty of the literature available. We hope that this publication will contribute to the evidence that the topic of supervision is one that is now undergoing an exciting phase of much more open investigation and conceptualization. These developments in supervision should lead to considerable benefits in the coming years for those who work in public health settings, where they are exposed to powerful psychological and emotional strains in themselves and their patients, as well as to those who offer formal psychotherapies in both public and private settings.

SUPERVISION AND ITS VICISSITUDES

CHAPTER ONE

On transference and countertransference and the technique of supervision

León Grinberg

Introduction

Among the many definitions that have been given to describe the process of supervision, I would like to underline the following ones: "It is a learning experience, in which an analyst is sharing with a colleague the fruits of clinical knowledge" (Arlow, 1963). Or, otherwise, "a complex process that takes place on behalf of an experienced analyst whose goal is to enable another analyst of lesser experience to be as efficient as possible in his task of helping the patient" (Horn, 1957). Supervision is a process that allows for personal and professional growth in the supervisee, and one of its objectives is to make it possible for the analytic situation to develop in a way that allows the supervisee to experience the phenomenon of psychoanalysis, to learn to conceptualize the experience he is living, and to reach and have insight in the experiences lived by the patient (Schlesinger, 1981).

John Keats (1817) referred to Negative Capability as that "when a man is capable of being in uncertainties, mystery, doubts, without any irritable reaching after facts and reason". I agree with

Blomfield (1985) when he says that analyst and supervisor should apply the principle of "negative capability" in psychoanalytic work. Our contact with early phantasies and primitive mental mechanisms, our accumulated knowledge, the application in therapy, in teaching, and in those theoretical branches all derive from the disciplined use of "negative capability".

As Frijling-Schreuder (1970) says: "It is convenient to create a 'working alliance' between the two members of the supervising experience so that the 'learning process' may develop under the best possible circumstances." This experience differs from the psychoanalytic situation as it does not stimulate regression. The supervisor and supervisee work together at an adult, sophisticated level. If anything, the supervisor offers himself implicitly as a model of identification. Possibly in the first phase the supervisee may begin with insecurity, dependence, or idealization, perhaps with an attitude of a certain opposition that will slowly be taken over by closer cooperation as insight and confidence increase. The respect for the clinical material is perhaps one of the most essential attitudes that should be transmitted to the supervisee.

Transference and countertransference in supervision

It is important to consider the myriad presentations of unconscious phantasy based on psychic reality that will appear in supervision as well as in the session that is being studied. There is also the possibility of some interference in the task of supervision due to transference and countertransference problems on behalf of the supervisee and supervisor.

The supervisor should examine very carefully his own prejudices, preferences, and susceptibilities in every case if he is to be able to stand aside from the personal battle that takes place between patient and therapist and keep a distance so as not to be involved in the anxiety and suffering determined by this conflict. One of his main functions would be to favour technical and personal development, while improving the "psychoanalytic instrument".

As to countertransference manifestations, both supervisor and supervisee should differentiate between those that are useful because they are a means of communication and valid technical instruments, and those that induce acting in and acting out in the supervisor or supervisee. Either of these would block the task and create serious problems in supervision.

Therapy or supervision of the countertransference

Supervisors often differ as to the attitude one should adopt with these countertransference problems of the supervisee with his patient. Should he discuss them with him? If so, when and how should he do so? These problems may become persistent or appear at a certain time with a greater intensity, distorting the development of the psychoanalytic process. Some authors maintain that it is preferable for the supervisor to help the student to discover the nature of his "involuntary participation" and to allow him to make conscious what stimuli he is responding to. But such an attitude brings back the discussion about the primary objective of supervision. Is it teaching or therapy? Other authors are definitely against adopting a therapeutic position in supervision involving an investigation of the countertransference of the supervisee.

Parallel process

A parallel process has been described that can develop between supervisee and patient, and between the supervisee and his supervisor, which implies that the student enacts towards the supervisor the same unconscious conflict that he has with his patient, or the patient with him. Some analysts say that, in some cases, the supervisor can help the student by sharing his countertransference with the supervisee.

EXAMPLES

A female supervisor relates the following case: a female supervisee, who is intelligent and had quite a good relationship with the supervisor, once brought some material of a borderline patient who was extremely destructive and had serious acting-out difficulties. The supervisee started the supervision session with a very astonishing sigh and later talked in a low voice and with apparent disinterest. The material was interesting, and the supervisor—against her usual style—found herself participating actively, suggesting different ideas to the supervisee. The supervisee listened without much enthusiasm, without making many comments. The supervisor felt uncomfortable and perceived in her countertransference feelings of helplessness. She realized then that such an active participation could have been a defence against that helplessness. She decided to tell the supervisee about these feelings, who in turn immediately responded saying that these were exactly the feelings she had felt with her patient. It seems that the patient had caused these feelings of helplessness in the therapist who had then induced them, through a parallel process, in the supervisor.

* * *

In this example, given by another female supervisor, the male supervisee had had a very strict upbringing. His female patient behaved in a very split manner in her life, showing a very rebellious attitude. The supervisee unconsciously colluded with (acted out) the rebellious side of his patient, which even affected the supervisee's work. The patient had been fired because she had rebelled against her boss. However, the supervisee had great difficulties in detecting the anxious and needy part of the patient. The supervisee did not respond when the supervisor pointed out his acting out with the patient. Yet he had a very kind and polite attitude towards the supervisor, asking about her health when the supervisor had flu, or about her holidays. The supervisor felt that she was reacting as a fragile person who needed to be reassured. This countertransference feeling allowed her to realize that the supervisee

> had split his relationship with the mother figure, acting considerately towards the "fragile mother" and encouraging his patient to act out her rebellious side (which coincided with that of the supervisee) towards the hated mother figure. She decided then to talk to the supervisee about his splitting and why it happened, so that he could become conscious that he was using it and modify his therapeutic attitude.

In my opinion, one could justify the supervisor's attitude in the first example because it was, from my point of view, a projective counteridentification (Grinberg, 1956, 1962, 1963, 1970, 1979, 1986, 1990), suffered by the therapist as a consequence of her patient's projective identifications, and she acted in a way that made the supervisor aware of her own feeling of helplessness. However, in the second example, the supervisor made a therapeutic intervention, interpreting the countertransference problem of the supervisee, which could lead to confusion of the supervisor's specific task and create a transference reaction that is not very appropriate to the setting and the task of supervision. I believe that she could have avoided it by simply pointing out that he was encouraging dissociation in the patient.

The supervisee's transference to the supervisor

The supervisee's transference to the supervisor has been discussed frequently. As I have said in publications and scientific meetings, it is possible that at the beginning of a clinical supervision the supervisee may deposit in the supervisor his ideal ego. Being incomplete is accepted, and for a while one idealizes somebody who is supposedly complete.

> The initial, idealised transference can be necessary and not a resistance; it can mean a moment of commitment that sustains the task. It is, however, appropriate that doubts, uncertainty and questioning appear somewhere along the line. Frustration at the differences between the imagined supervisor and the real supervisor, must be experienced so that the development

> of the process will continue. Development will stop when the supervisee is fixed in an idealised transference. The supervisee risks becoming an echo of the supervisor, losing his own developing identity as an analyst and becoming a mere clone of the supervisor, negating his capacity to think and to create. [Casullo & Resnizky, 1993]

The supervisor's transference and parallel process

I consider it useful, nevertheless, to think about the supervisor's transference towards the supervisee, which has been much less written about in the psychoanalytic literature. Undoubtedly, as I state later, the supervisor cannot be an outsider to his own emotional reactions that appear in relation to the supervisee whom he must teach and evaluate. I have referred above to the parallel process that can lead the supervisee to repeat actively in supervision what he has suffered passively with his patient. Sometimes these repetitions are real "actings-in" and produce specific responses in the supervisor. In this case one must investigate the relationship that exists between supervisor and supervisee in the "here and now" of the supervision and not try to capture the transference of the patient through the material the supervisee brings, as it can be distorted. The transference–countertransference relationship between supervisee and patient sometimes becomes present in a displaced way during supervision. The supervisee can revive with the supervisor some of the experiences that he has lived through with the patient and enact them, making the supervisor feel what he has felt with the patient. Some authors have considered the parallel process as something that can be used by the supervisor as a resistance to deny his own transference. This idea is supported by Barbara Stimmel (1995). She insists that the sophisticated concept of parallel process is used by the supervisor, on many occasions, to avoid becoming conscious of his transference towards the supervisee; this transference would be independent of the problems of the case that is being presented.

Example

> One of the examples Stimmel wrote about was the case of a resident therapist who during supervision manifested certain persistent doubts about the supervisor's capacity to maintain confidentiality. The supervisor was part of the administration in the institution, with which the supervisee's patient also had links. It seems that the resident therapist had identified with the patient's resistance to express herself freely in the analysis because of the lack of confidence in the therapist's discretion. The frustration experienced by the supervisor because of the supervisee's attitude mirrored the frustration of the supervisee with his patient in such a way that the supervisor "interpreted" the parallel process, and this apparently removed the "impasse". Shortly afterwards the therapist asked if the supervisor would take care of this patient in the future when he finished his training. It was only then that the supervisor realized that her feelings towards the supervisee were protective, affectionate, and warm. The independent parallel process had diverted attention from the fact that the supervision was being conducted partly from within the framework of a positive/mother–son transference.

So it seems that the parallel process is a dynamic phenomenon that in specific circumstances can offer the supervisor protection against awareness of either certain gratifications or thoughts that might make him ashamed or of rejected phantasy towards the therapist. The parallel process is useful and can give helpful information sometimes, but it also becomes a convenient area for hiding undesirable transferences of the supervisor. I personally think that these transferences are not as completely independent as Barbara Stimmel indicates. It is my belief that it is always the supervisee's direct or indirect participation or his patient's material that stimulates the development of these transferences.

Psychoanalytic knowledge

It has been said that the supervisor should have the capacity to transmit psychoanalytic knowledge, not because he is more knowledgeable but because he knows it in a different way. Therefore, some authors maintain that one can help the supervisee to understand his patient better through some of his countertransference manifestations. This would not be asking the supervisor to function as the student's analyst or trying to make him confront unconscious personal conflicts. Of course, he must always respect the setting of the supervision and keep a correct distance between himself and the supervisee (Haesler, 1993). He must function in a way that is not intrusive, trying to take advantage of countertransference responses that can be as specific as phenomena that are the echo of the patient's material.

Terttu Eskelinen de Folch (1981) writes that sometimes she asks the supervisee about the content of his feelings, searching to know better the quality of transference–countertransference experiences. She considers it important to teach the supervisee to observe his emotional reactions, to verbalize them to himself, and to be able to talk about them to the supervisor. In her opinion, focusing attention on the supervisee's countertransference is a means of understanding the patient's transference. As an example, she states that, if a patient threatens to commit suicide, the supervisor can only realize whether this is something serious or not if she knows the supervisee's emotional response. However, one cannot forget about the risks of this technical attitude in stepping over the boundaries between the supervisor's function and the therapist's function. This area needs to be open to considerable debate.

Some supervisors maintain that the "teaching–learning alliance" is a greenhouse plant that should be specially taken care of and nurtured. But if the supervisee has the minimum conditions for analysis and intellectual capacity, and the supervisor does not interfere too much, the teaching situation will develop in a natural way. In any case, the supervisor has the responsibility to check whether the evolution of the learning task is not as good as it should be, and to decide what should be done to improve it. One of the problems to be taken into account is the supervisee's countertransference to his patient or to the supervisor.

Schlesinger (1981) maintains that minor countertransference reactions of the supervisee are almost inevitable, but if they are persistent and important they can distort the development of the analytic situation. In these cases, if the supervisee is not in analysis, he suggests that the supervisor should help him to discover the nature of his "involuntary participation" and the effect it is producing on his patient. The supervisor who feels the need to enter into an area that involves the supervisee's countertransference should begin by adopting the working hypothesis that the supervisee's difficulty could be a product of his lack of knowledge. For Schlesinger, it is only when the supervisee proves incapable of using the knowledge as to what is interfering in his capacity as an analyst that the supervisor can point out the dynamic factors in the supervisee's personality.

Other sorts of problems are related to the supervisee's and supervisor's personalities as well as different styles, as we will see in the following pages.

The setting for supervision

Supervisory situations, like psychoanalytic treatment, call for an appropriate setting (Grinberg, 1970). I understand "setting" to be an adherence to a set of given behaviour patterns so that the task can be accomplished under optimum conditions, without being interfered with by attitudes on either side that may endanger the task. To understand better what, in supervision, this setting consists of, I could define it by stating its opposite: supervision is not, and must not be, therapy. The setting must be such as to make explicit the difference between therapy and supervision. One of the problems that could appear is that the supervisee, unconsciously, and for various reasons, can look to the supervisor to act as a therapist. This request is sometimes a response to a need to satisfy a transference dissociation, reviving an "idealized analyst" and projecting the "persecutory image" into his training analyst, or vice versa. The supervisor should take precautions to avoid contingencies of this sort and will achieve his goal if he keeps strictly to the setting of supervision. It is helpful, therefore, for every encounter between supervisor and supervisee to begin with a brief chat, so that the relationship that is established is clearly between colleagues, without, of course, becoming too familiar and interfering with the specific task.

Turning briefly to a technical aspect of supervision, I would like to point out a fact that seems quite meaningful to me, one that I have repeatedly observed (Grinberg, 1986). It is quite common for students to begin supervision with a trivial comment about the weather, or some delay that they had suffered because of traffic, or an experience that happened at the seminar, a family episode concerning their children, and so forth. Experience has taught me that these incidental comments are often valuable as a kind of free association indirectly connected with the main theme of the patient's material that has been brought to the supervision. Unconsciously, the students were able to take in latent and fundamental aspects of the material that they could not grasp in a manifest way. Making the situation more explicit whenever it happens will allow supervisees to acquire more confidence in themselves and to dare to handle the content more directly.

Problems of supervisees

Supervising has been, and still is, very gratifying to me because of the mutual benefits that flow from the common investigation of the two parties and because of the interest, receptiveness, and constant stimulus that I have always received from my younger colleagues. However, in some cases I have had to confront some problems derived from certain personalities or characteristics of the transference of some students and their peculiar attitude to supervision.

When confronted with the persecutory anxiety that supervision can awaken, some supervisees resort to manic attitudes, pretending that they have understood everything that the patient has brought in. It then becomes important to point out systematically the mistakes they have made because of their misunderstanding and the inherent difficulties of the clinical material that has been presented. Other supervisees, on the other hand, react with strong inhibitions, which makes it very difficult for them to accomplish the minimum required. They tend to repress what they have understood in the material and, as a rule, their interpretations are scanty and ambiguous. These are, of course, two extreme positions: there is a whole spectrum of intermediate attitudes between them.

I would now like to refer, in a more specific way, to the transference problems determined by those students whose personalities have more severe pathologies and which have negative influences on the relationship with the supervisor and the development of the supervisory process.

It may happen that some exceedingly greedy personalities go to supervision not to learn but to grasp and store up whatever knowledge they may receive, without discrimination. They admire and envy the supervisor's capacity, experience, and cleverness but do not try to assimilate his teachings; instead, they try to "swallow" him so that they may become the absolute owners of what he possesses. In other cases, envy can be so regressive that they cannot stand the other person having knowledge that they lack, and therefore they try to destroy the supervisor through insidious attacks. They may behave with an extremely critical attitude, objecting to the supervisor's ideas and systematically disqualifying his work, castrating his mental capacity. This situation becomes even worse when the competitiveness and rivalry become more acute, to the extent that the supervisee tries to dazzle his supervisor omnipotently with his supposed "intelligence" and show of superiority. Whenever the supervisor tries to include a technical suggestion, the supervisee reacts saying: "Of course, I have already done what you suggest."

Sometimes they improvise or invent interpretations that were not really said in the context of the session. They base them on their supervisor's comments, transforming them into their "own interpretation", or try to explain them in the following way: "What a coincidence, that is exactly what I said in the following sequence of the session, with almost the same words you have just used."

I have mentioned the student who lies. It is important to consider not only how serious and frequent this symptom may be, but also the different reasons why it can happen. Some students, with a different reaction to persecution, fear being invaded by the supervisor's teaching or feel that they have to obey and incorporate the supervisor's point of view and ways of working, which may differ from their own style. They fear supervision as a possible threat to their identity and defend themselves by talking all the time or reading endless sessions, so that the supervisor can participate as little as possible. The opposite phenomenon takes place in those supervisees who choose their worst cases, with the greatest difficulties, and those who have manifestly analysed wrongly. I am not referring to wanting to take to supervision problem cases for help in overcoming the difficulties of the analysis: this is obviously normal and is one of the aims of supervision. I am thinking of those supervisees with a marked masochistic tendency who "need" to show their errors and the most negative side of their work. They sometimes exaggerate the defects and can even distort the material. They lie, not to look good but, paradoxically, to make themselves look worse than they are. This may be due, amongst other reasons, to guilt feelings and a need for punishment because of rivalry and competitiveness, not only towards the supervisor but also towards their peers and their own analyst as well.

Problems of supervisors

Supervisors do not have all their neurotic conflicts completely resolved either. These conflicts can be reactivated and become more intense, especially in certain circumstances, such as when certain countertransference feelings are experienced in the supervisory situation.

The supervisor may have a tendency to seek discussion and debate with the supervisee on subjects well outside the specific aim of the teaching–learning relationship, due perhaps to the analyst's isolated activity during most of the day and minimum contact with the extra-analytic world. This isolation, and the regression it brings about, may provoke a greater need to exchange personal information.

A supervisor with paranoid characteristics may have to face serious problems in performing his function. He can be afraid that the supervisee may want to deprive him of his original ideas and will try to teach in a very cautious way, giving as little of himself as possible, and restricting his comments to general concepts. Obviously, the supervision that takes place in such an atmosphere is bound to be vitiated; it will lack an essential aspect of the teaching, which consists precisely in the capacity of the teacher to transmit his wide and deep experience. It may happen that this paranoid tendency can take place in analysts who, for different reasons, have difficulties in writing, developing their concepts, and publishing their work. They are usually intelligent people, with a potential capacity for teaching fruitfully, but because of these specific problems may accuse others of having taken their ideas and of presenting them as their own. Any teacher, and therefore any supervisor, should be fully aware of this problem and work it through constructively.

There can be the opposite situation: that of the supervisor with a depressive personality, and with a masochistic tendency in his work. Owing to conflictual phantasies related to guilt feelings, this sort of supervisor will try to be tremendously generous and compulsively pour out everything he knows and possesses. It will be difficult for him to draw a line between the number of ideas he "needs" to transmit and overwhelming the student with an avalanche of knowledge. Of course, I could describe other manifestations of a supervisor's psychopathology and the various emotional reactions when faced with the supervisee or the clinical material that he reports. Nobody is exempt from these reactions, and it is important to be alert and to be able to detect them when they appear and prevent them from affecting the process of supervision. What is desirable in the specific relationship between teacher and student is what Erikson (1963) called "generativity"—that is to say, "the capacity to generate interest in establishing and guiding the next generation".

I will now refer to the experience that took place several years ago in the Argentine Psychoanalytic Association with young analysts, consisting of several meetings under the general title of "Dialogue with a Group of Psychoanalysts about the Theory and Technique of Supervision". The objective was to confront the problems and experience of supervision from all possible theoretical and technical points of view. This experience was tremendously useful and very stimulating both for the colleagues who participated and for me. As the "Dialogues" had been recorded, I was able to transcribe them in my book, *La Supervisión Psicoanalítica:*

Teoría y Práctica [Psychoanalytic Supervision: Theory and Practice] (1986).

I find it convenient to reproduce briefly some of the interventions and my answers, because they are related to what we are discussing now:

Question: "I would like to ask a question about the interaction between supervisor and supervisee. What must we do when the supervisee replies to what the supervisor said with an 'Oh yes, but what you have said is what I interpreted later'? An answer like that establishes a sort of interaction which, at least for me, is difficult because perhaps the supervisee has not realized that he is beginning to compete with the supervisor and is, in a certain way, attacking the normal relationship between both of them. I would like to know how this sort of problem can be resolved."

Answer: "There can be pathology, both in supervisor and supervisee. It is very important to differentiate the situations, which are sometimes unavoidable, of competitiveness and rivalry and to try to clean the working field of this sort of contamination. In general, I do not tell the supervisee that his attitude is due to a competitive situation with me, but I try to solve this by inviting him to think together with me about his comments. I consider that the most important thing to teach is how to think, so that they can think on their own."

Question: "So you, as a supervisor, find yourself inhibited from using the instrument of the therapeutic situation and operate a different instrument in supervision?"

Answer: "I do think that there is a different instrument in supervision that must be used in the right way with patience and tolerance. When there is an evident discrepancy I try to handle the situation accepting their point of view and asking them to put it alongside mine. I try to show them a way of looking at the material from a different perspective. Sometimes they are right and I accept their point of view, others are very stubborn and wrong. When the situation is very difficult, I tell them that they need to base their statements on clinical material."

Question: "I would like to refer to another problem, which is related to the difference of trends of thought between supervisor and supervisee. To what extent can this produce conflicts?"

Answer: "I have never had any trouble in that sense. Sometimes, I have even felt it has a certain advantage, preventing the risk of submission to a certain line of thought sustained by the supervisor. I am convinced that there is enormous benefit to be derived from confronting different frames of reference, when it can be done without dogmatism or persecution. I do not discard the realization that sometimes when there is a predominance of persecutory anxieties in the supervisee, this can be channelled through the phantasy of defending his theory blindly. There can then be serious difficulties in the common task, and it is very important to make the situation as clear as possible, very cautiously. I clarify that supervision is not something intended to attack a specific theory but is there to clarify the meaning of the clinical material that has been brought, and that this can be done from different perspectives. I must underline the usefulness to the student of having at least two supervisions, so that he can learn and confront different styles. Sometimes it can happen that he can identify predominantly with one of the styles until he filters his own technique and finally finds his own style."

Question: "I will ask a question that involves the whole philosophy about the purpose of supervision: When does it end?"

Answer: "This is also a very interesting question. There are students who ask to continue supervision after the official period of time established by the institute for analytic training. Sometimes this is based on a desire to learn in more depth and breadth about analytic work and to receive supervision on other patients. Other supervisees prefer to stick to the official time and do not continue supervision. Some people end because they wish to go on to another supervisor. This is very understandable and should be accepted. Others are in a hurry to finish their training as soon as possible and stick to the formal setting without showing any more interest in learning itself. On the pretext of fear of interminable analysis (theoretically a possibility, but rare in practice), some analysts may ally with their patient's resistance and interrupt analysis prematurely without sufficient working through, leading to bad endings. I think the contrary: that it is appropriate to exhaust all possibilities and allow the analytic process to work itself through thoroughly, leading to an appropriate ending. The same can be said of supervision.

"Following a parallel with analysis, I would say that, in the same way as we try to help the patient to acquire a capacity for self-analysis, it is also our task as supervisors to allow the supervisees to learn not only a technique and a method, but also to be able to supervise their own work and be able to confront and solve urgent problems in their patient's analysis, to recognize mistakes and be able to rectify them. I think that these would be the basic conditions for one to be able to talk about the end of supervision. I do not exclude the possibility that after some time there can be a further experience of supervision, just as there can be a reanalysis."

Countertransference and projective counteridentification

I would like to come back to the important problem of the supervisor's attitude to the supervisee's countertransference to his patient. This is a subject that has been discussed in a number of scientific meetings and papers (Arlow, 1963; Blomfield, 1985; DeBell, 1963; Fleming & Benedek, 1966; Lebovici, 1970; Solnit, 1970).

A descriptive and comprehensive approach to the countertransference phenomenon has been described lately by Bouchard, Normandin, and Séguin (1995). They write about three types of mental activity:

- an objective-rational attitude, referring to a method of observation that is non-defensive;

- a reactive mental state that corresponds to the classic notion of unconscious countertransference as an obstacle and defence;
- the reflective attitude that involves a pre-conscious and conscious activity. The latter takes place thanks to objective observation of our subjectiveness and countertransference.

I would like to differentiate between two large categories within countertransference problems. One corresponds to the problems of countertransference itself, and the other concerns what I have called "projective counteridentification" (Grinberg, 1956). The latter is a specific phenomenon and different from countertransference, because it is precipitated by the patient and determined by the quality and intensity of his projective-identification mechanisms.

In projective counteridentification, the analyst may have the feeling of being no longer himself and of unavoidably becoming transformed into the object that the patient, unconsciously, wanted him to be (id, ego, or some internal object), or to experience those affects (anger, depression, anxiety, boredom, etc.) the analysand has forced into him. Even if the situation prevails only for a short time, the analyst will resort to all kinds of rationalizations to justify his feelings of bewilderment.

The analyst is affected to the extent that he feels induced to experience emotions and to act the roles that the patient has, unconsciously, projected into him. The analyst will then react as if he had "concretely and actually" incorporated and assimilated the aspects projected into him, and sometimes he will allow himself to be manipulated by them.

I have often been asked about the difference between countertransference and projective counteridentification. To summarize, I would say that through countertransference each analyst can identify with the internal objects of the patient or react in a particular manner according to the nature of his own conflicts. In contrast, in projective-counteridentification reactions, the affects contained in the analysand's projective identification will predominate in the analyst. To clarify this difference further, I would say that different analysts because of their countertransference will react in a different way to the material of a hypothetical patient. This same patient in another phase of the analysis with different analysts would bring about almost the same emotional response in all of them because of the use at that moment of a specific type of projective identification from the patient.

Giovacchini (1990) mentions the case of a patient who caused him great irritation, without his being able to understand why. He had the idea of recording a session, with the patient's permission, and a short time later he played it back to a group of colleagues and students, without previously informing them of his problem. To his surprise, all the listeners experienced a similar irritation to his own; that is, the patient was producing the same reaction of projective counteridentification in different people.

I published my first paper on projective counteridentification in 1956. I was happy when I found confirmation of my ideas in Bion's book, *Learning from Experience* (1962), in which he remarked that: "The theory of countertransferences offers only partly satisfactory explanation because it is concerned with the manifestation as a symptom of the analyst's unconscious motives and therefore it *leaves the patient's contribution unexplained*" (p. 24; my italics). So, Bion also accepts the emergence of emotions in the analyst produced by the patient (through his projective counteridentification) and which are independent, up to a certain point, of the countertransference of the analyst. According to my point of view, both countertransference and projective-counteridentification reactions can co-exist, with one predominating over the other, depending on the level of the patient's regression and the content of the clinical material.

I believe it is fundamental for the supervisor to differentiate between these two categories every time he is confronted with this sort of problem, because the countertransference aspects should be solved in the supervisee's analysis and projective counteridentification must be tackled in a more specific way during supervision. When the student has difficulties or blind spots that are predominantly due to a situation or conflict of his own, which are within the area of countertransference itself, the supervisor may refrain from making a direct remark, but he can point out that there is a difficulty and show how to approach the dynamics of what is happening to the patient. Some authors think that it is better to make the situation explicit and advise that the student should try to see in his analysis what has happened. But this procedure is questioned by others, as it may have an unnecessarily disturbing effect on the supervisee.

I wish to dwell on the issue of projective counteridentification because this belongs to the realm of supervision. The supervisor must apply himself to the difficulties arising from this situation, since it is in this area that he can help the student to realize the conflict or technical error that is not always conscious to him. These difficulties are generally determined by the patient inducing the therapist—through the use of projective identification—to act a certain role and to assume certain special attitudes or to experience certain emotions.

The supervisor will be most helpful when he is able to use his experience and knowledge of the existence of the projective-counteridentification reaction to differentiate when the analyst/student is under the effect of projective counteridentification from when he is experiencing a personal neurotic difficulty. The supervisor will have the clinical material that will show the source of this disturbance, and using the material he must show the student where and why this projective-counteridentification reaction took place.

The student, in turn, can make the supervisor feel the same emotional reaction that the patient has made him feel. As I said earlier, this would be a parallel process. If the supervisor is able to make conscious the genesis of his own affective response, then he will be able to show the supervisee, from a more objective and experienced point of view, the origin of his emotional reaction in the session with his patient.

Other frameworks for the same phenomena

There have been authors who have referred to similar problems using different theoretical frameworks, and consequently they use a different terminology to conceptualize and describe the phenomenon. I believe that many disagreements are due to semantic rather than conceptual reasons. Arlow (1963) says, in reference to this kind of phenomenon, that the therapist shifts from the role of reporting the experience he has had with his patient to "experiencing" his patient's experience; that is to say, the supervisor may find evidence that the supervisee "acts" an identification with his patient. In a fragment of the material of one of her patients, Betty Joseph (1988) says: "I could understand the way in which I was being pushed and taken to feel and react. . . . N was invading me with desperation and at the same time trying to force me unconsciously to keep calm." Sandler and Sandler (1978) refer to the attempts of the patient to manipulate the analyst in order to evoke a specific sort of response in him. To Hanna Segal (1981), "there is a whole area of the patient's pathology that is directed specifically to disturb the situation of containment of the analysis, using invasion of the analyst's mind in a seductive and aggressive way, creating confusion and anxiety in him".

I think that projective counteridentification is not only a disturbance. On the contrary, I believe it can also be a starting point to experiencing a spectrum of emotions, which, well understood and sublimated, may be turned into a very important technical instrument to enter into contact with the deepest levels of the analysands' material. The concept is useful not only for the analyst, but also for the supervisor when he experiences projective counteridentification.

Examples

A student started his session of supervision saying that he felt depressed and in a bad mood. As this was something unusual and as I thought that this was a personal situation, I preferred not to make any comments and suggested we should go on to the material of the session we were discussing. He said that this time he had had difficulties in writing down the last session, and he was afraid that he had forgotten some sequences. He complained that the lack of time did not allow him to do everything he should and that was why he had not been able to take notes of the session of that week, as he had wanted to. He then said that he felt hot, and he asked me if I could open the window (it was a cool autumn day). I must admit that I also started to feel hot. I was half surprised and found it quite strange. I insisted on looking at the material, suspecting some connection with it. It was a claustrophobic female patient, who was usually depressed and often complained of a serious conflict in her marriage. She usually reproached her husband because of his manic personality and because he was aggressive. This time the patient had come to her session completely "different", according to the supervisee's own expression. She had never been so manic and talked so much, and he had felt "attacked" by her. It was not difficult to show him that the patient "had identified with the aggressive husband" and had behaved in a totally manic and aggressive way just as the husband did. At the same time, she had projected into the therapist her own depressive, complaining, claustrophobic part, and he needed to act this out during the supervision, projecting into me part of what the patient had deposited into him.

* * *

A supervisor, while listening to the material of the session of a borderline patient that a quite experienced student was reading to him, started to feel sleepy, and this got worse as the student went on reading. He could not recognize any personal motivation that would justify this sleepiness, as he had not felt tired before the supervision. On the other hand, his relationship with the student was very cordial, and he liked the student because of his capacity to work, his receptivity, and his capacity to assimilate the points made by the supervisor. He could attribute his sleepiness neither to the tone with which the student was reading the material, as he did not think it was monotonous, nor to the contents, because it was an interesting session of a new patient who had only a short time ago started treatment. Given the good relationship he had with the student, he decided to tell him what was happening. The student, in turn, reacted in a very interested way, saying that he had felt something similar with the patient during several sessions. He, too, had had to fight his desire to sleep, and precisely in the middle of the session that he was reading to the supervisor he had fallen asleep. It seems that the student, in using projective identification, needed to provoke in the supervisor that which the patient had projected into him as a way of transmitting this specific technical problem; in this way, the supervisor could help him to solve it.

* * *

When receiving a supervisee who was coming to his supervision session, I was struck because when he greeted me he did not shake hands as usual. He was quite anxious and worried and said that he wanted to tell me what had happened in one of his sessions with a patient. He had felt very moved when the patient told him that her son had had an operation: her little boy's arm had been amputated because of an accident. At a certain point, the patient cried with despair and extended her hand backwards towards the analyst. The analyst realized that he had not been able to relieve her with his interpretations and felt compelled to respond with a gesture towards the woman; he felt it to be a desperate demand for help, and he took her hand and held it. Then he was quite shocked and felt guilty because of this and admitted that he felt uncomfortable towards me because of the technical transgression he had committed. I pointed out then that he had not shaken hands with me when he arrived. He was very surprised, because he had not noticed this at a conscious level, and then he remembered that the patient had not shaken hands when she had arrived either. He doubted whether it was convenient to include this in the interpretation but then he repressed it. Studying the material, we were able to realize that the woman's gesture not only corresponded to asking for help, but, having projected into the therapist the image of her son, she was trying magically to cancel the painful reality of an unconscious phantasy in which her analyst/son still had his arm and was able to shake her hand. The therapist unconsciously counteridentified with this phantasy and acted the role. When he came to supervision, the student unconsciously tried to cancel his action in the session with his behaviour of not shaking my hand, but also reproduced with another acting-out his counteridentification with the patient, who had not shaken his hand when she arrived in the session.

Concluding remarks

To end this chapter, I would like to point out that if we try to cover everything that happens in a session of supervision, then, because there are so many contingencies related to transference and countertransference problems, we will find that there are many possible sources of conflict for both the direct participants—supervisor and supervisee—as well as people behind the scenes, such as the training analysts, the other supervisor, the institute, and so forth.

I therefore think it necessary to spell out the need to respect the internal temporal process for each supervisee as a priority in the learning process of supervision. In this sense, my attitude in the first period of work with a new supervisee is to transmit information at a certain pace, and not to be in a hurry to show my specific ways of confronting clinical material. I try to get to know the way in which the supervisee works and what his main difficulties are, and to help him to correct certain mistakes in the way he understands the material and concepts, and so on. Gradually, I start to introduce my own point of view, always based on the clinical material. On the other hand, I try to make it explicit to the supervisee that we are working with material that belongs to the past—that is, experiences of sessions that have already happened—and that they will probably have nothing to do with the next day's session. I also underline that it is useful for the supervisee to have a working hypothesis, without implying that this should be immediately transformed into interpretations. I also insist, for the benefit of understanding as clearly as possible, that I be provided with the manifest contents of sessional material. If there is anything obscure or confusing, I ask questions to clarify as much as possible.

As I wrote earlier, supervision is a very encouraging activity for both supervisor and supervisee, because it offers a new field of observation. It promotes thinking, learning, and the correcting of ideas. One constantly rediscovers the unconscious, the many phenomena of transference, countertransference, and projective counteridentification, which all lead to the asking of more and more questions. All analysts and supervisors, to a greater or lesser degree, go through a process of change through their receptiveness to new ideas in the activity of supervision. The capacity to revitalize oneself constantly is one that we should transmit to our young colleagues.

CHAPTER TWO

Psychoanalytic supervision of untrained therapists

Victor Sedlak

Introduction

In this chapter I describe aspects of the supervision of therapists who have not had a formal, comprehensive training, part of which would have included psychoanalysis for themselves. I argue that the supervisory process with such people throws light upon several important aspects of all psychoanalytic supervision. Principally, I wish to show that a therapist's work will deteriorate at the moment at which he is unable to deal with the countertransference in a professional, psychoanalytic manner. More specifically, it is when a negative countertransference is being experienced and cannot be managed that problems most frequently arise. This can be a greater handicap to the therapist and pose a greater risk to the therapeutic endeavour than the therapist's lack of knowledge of the finer points of the theory of psychoanalysis.

A longer version of this chapter was given at the Second International Conference of the European Federation for Psychoanalytic Psychotherapy in Toledo, Spain, May/June 1996.

The unavailability of personal therapy or analysis and of a good training experience does not stop people in the caring professions working in what they consider to be an analytic or dynamic way. Senior practitioners can of course choose to have little to do with this possible diminution of standards; alternatively they can explore in what ways they can help, while maintaining their professional integrity. I have chosen the latter course.

This chapter is based largely on my work supervising therapists in Leeds, a large city in the north of England, where for a number of years I was the only analyst. My views are also influenced by my frequent visits to Warsaw to provide teaching and supervision to members of the Polish Society for the Development of Psychoanalysis. In each of these settings I have taught and supervised mental health professionals who have taken a very serious interest in psychoanalysis and psychoanalytic psychotherapy without having been able to complete official trainings. Typically, they are well read and have attended many workshops and training events but lack the experience of an integrated and disciplined programme specifically designed to equip them to do psychoanalytic psychotherapy.

Psychoanalytic psychotherapy is a branch of knowledge having its own rules of conduct and understanding—or technique and theory, as these are most usually described. In order to acquire such a discipline one requires a training that transmits knowledge of the principles of that discipline, via seminars, organized reading, teaching, and so on. However, with the disciplines of psychoanalysis and psychoanalytic psychotherapy there is an emotional element to the work, and training therefore includes the component of personal analysis or therapy to help students acquire an emotional range and resilience. This allows practitioners to apply the theoretical principles of the discipline in their therapeutic work. Great stress is placed upon this because of the belief that a psychoanalytic experience will centre around an emotional relationship and that this will stir up personal feelings in the therapist. Unless these can be dealt with in a professional manner, and this is indeed difficult since the countertransference is in the main an unconscious response, then the therapist will be unable to apply his knowledge of the principles of psychoanalysis in a therapeutic fashion.

Jacobs, David, and Meyer (1995) describe succinctly the capacities needed to use the countertransference: "to contain, to identify and finally to analyse or relate the internal affective experience (of the therapist) to the current (clinical) situation." Such emotional and cognitive work on the part of the therapist allows a psychoanalytic activity—that is, the translation of emotional forces into meaningful words—to continue. A failure to do such synthesizing will lead to acting in, acting out, and failures of understanding and therapeutic endeavour.

There are many reasons why a reasonably successful personal analysis or therapy is central to enabling a practitioner to function better as a therapist. My focus here is on two of these: the way in which a therapeutic experience will allow the personality to be more tolerant of external reality, and, the manner in which it promotes greater acceptance of internal reality. A good analytic experience will lessen a person's need to use omnipotent and omniscient ways of perceiving the world, and it will decrease the confusion between the actual external world and its distortions by projection. Furthermore, a good analytic experience will enable the person to develop sufficient emotional range and resilience to be able to bear and to accommodate to the difficulties thrown up by external reality. In addition, and very much connected to this, there will be a lessening of the pathological aspects of a punitive superego that does not allow the person to tolerate his thoughts and affects. Both of these developments are crucial to work in which the therapist needs to perceive reasonably accurately the actual state of the patient and then be able to allow and monitor his own emotional reaction to that state.

In order to clarify further the nature of psychoanalytic activity and the difficult emotional work that it involves, I go back to Freud and to the beginning of a period of his work that gave psychoanalysis some extremely important conceptual tools. This also provides an early example of an analysis ending prematurely, and probably unsatisfactorily, because of the therapist's countertransferential difficulties.

Freud and the Wolf Man

In his technical paper "Remembering, Repeating and Working Through," written in 1914, Freud first introduced the concept of the repetition compulsion. Although he did not view this phenomenon as the destructive activity that he would later come to see it, he does offer advice about the technique of dealing with the more obdurate and stubborn manifestations of a patient's problems (which can be read as Freud acting as a supervisor using the theoretical concepts available to him in 1914):

> The first step in overcoming the resistances is made, as we know, by the analyst's uncovering the resistance, which is never recognised by the patient, and acquainting him with it. Now it seems that beginners in analytic practice are inclined to look on this introductory step as constituting the whole of their work. I have often been asked to advise upon cases in which the doctor complained that he had pointed out his resistance to the patient and that nevertheless no change had set in; indeed, the resistance had become all the stronger, and the whole situation was more obscure than ever. The treatment seemed to make no headway. This gloomy foreboding always proved mistaken. The treatment was as a rule progressing most satisfactorily. . . . One must allow the patient time to become conversant with this resistance with which he has now become acquainted, to work through it, to overcome it, by continuing, in defiance of it, the analytic work according to the fundamental rule of analysis. . . . The doctor has nothing else to do than to wait and let things take their course, a course which cannot be avoided nor always hastened. If he holds fast to this conviction he will often be spared the illusion of having failed when in fact he is conducting the treatment on the right lines. [Freud, 1914, p. 155]

This was a very clear statement of the need to *keep analysing* and not to abandon the task of trying to understand what is going on in the consulting room. In other words, Freud advocated that the therapist kept to the discipline of psychoanalysis and resisted the temptation to become eclectic. However, it was also a very optimistic view of the knowledge base of psychoanalysis as it was in 1914: "Just keep on as you are, youngster, it will be all right", Freud seemed to be saying. He implied that the nature of the repressed instinctual impulses that fed the resistance were already known in 1914 and that the analyst simply had to continue to apply this knowledge. Yet this was not the case, and Freud knew this because in his consulting room he had been unable to follow his own advice.

In the middle of 1914 Freud had done something that was completely counter to the counsel quoted above. At that time he was in the fourth year of the Wolf Man's analysis, and

> . . . its difficulties were more conspicuous than its fruitfulness. "The first years of the treatment brought scarcely any change." The Wolf Man was courtesy itself but kept himself "unassailably entrenched" in an attitude of "submissive indifference. He listened, understood, and permitted nothing to touch him." Freud found it all very frustrating. The Wolf Man's "unimpeachable intelligence was as if cut off from the instinctual forces that governed his conduct." The Wolf Man took untold months before he began to participate in the work of the analysis; and then, once he felt the pressure of internal change, he resumed his gently sabotaging ways. In this predicament, Freud decided to set a termination date—one year hence—for the analysis, and stick to it inflexibly. [Gay, 1988, p. 291]

Freud did not have available to him the contemporary understanding of the countertransference. He did not consider that the setting of a termination date as a means of spurring the patient to make use of the analysis was an acting-in on his behalf. He did give us a clue, however, to what one aspect of his countertransference may have been. In advocating the technique of setting a termination date, he insisted that, once set, it could not be changed, and he quoted the saying "The lion only springs once". This surely informs us that the Wolf Man's subtle but constant negative therapeutic reactions had got under Freud's skin; the saying certainly suggests he felt murderous towards his patient. It was not that Freud was put off by direct expressions of aggression; in a letter to Ferenczi written after his initial consultation with the Wolf Man, he noted with pleasure that this new patient was an interesting case who disclosed in the first hour that he thought Freud to be a "Jewish swindler" and that he already entertained thoughts of "shitting on his analyst's head" (Gay, 1988, p. 287). This conscious verbalization of his patient's aggression did not perturb Freud;

what finally undid Freud's resolve to do as he advised others to do, that is, keep on analysing, was the constant repudiation of his work—one might say, the daily shitting on his head by the Wolf Man. I think this is a good example of the silent way in which the negative therapeutic reaction is so often expressed and of the fact that a therapist who is able to tolerate overt expressions of aggression can be undone by a covert silent resistance.

I have suggested that Freud was unable to help the Wolf Man beyond a certain point, but there is also a way that he did keep to his discipline in that he continued to try to clarify the dynamic factors that lay beneath such clinical presentations. The body of work that Freud produced in the decade following 1914 allows a much more comprehensive understanding of the *anti-developmental factors* in the human mind which mitigate against growth and which so frequently produce negative countertransferential reactions. In this period, Freud introduced the concepts of narcissism and melancholia; there was further thinking on the problem of masochism; he described the concept of the death instinct and he discovered the superego and its melancholic and pathological manifestations. All these discoveries enable practitioners now to understand, in a way that Freud did not in 1914, the complex pathology of destructive narcissism that underlay the Wolf Man's presentation. There is now a far better comprehension of some of the most pathological manifestations of the repetition compulsion, of how they exhibit themselves in object relations, internal and external, and of the pervasive hold that these factors can have on the human mind.

The repetition compulsion, countertransference, and contemporary psychotherapy

There are a number of reasons why this history is important and pertinent to the topic of supervision, and particularly to the supervision of untrained therapists. In the United Kingdom at least, but probably in all developed countries, the last thirty years have seen a great spread of the availability of counselling and of many different forms of psychotherapy. Many more patients are being treated by psychotherapeutic means; a large number of these patients, particularly those seen in the public sector, are very damaged individuals. It is mainly a borderline or even psychotic population that is increasingly referred to psychology, psychiatry, and psychotherapy departments in the public sector. That is to say, such departments are increasingly treating a population in which anti-developmental forces of the human mind have their most pervasive hold. The need of these departments to attract funding also plays a part in them offering treatment to these patients.

There has not been a corresponding increase in the provision of training in psychotherapy for mental health professionals, and it is also the case that, in most public sector services, patients are actually treated by the least experienced members of staff. Thus, patients whose problems are such that they are prone to negative therapeutic reactions—and hence to producing negative countertransferential responses—are often being treated by therapists who are not specifically equipped by their professional training to manage their countertransference in a professional way. This leads to many problems such as therapists' despair, professional burnout, sadistic (usually unconscious) treatment of patients, talented therapists choosing to move away from the public to the private sector or into management, and many other such manifestations. Can psychoanalytic supervision help in this dilemma and, if so, in what way? In order to address this question, I present some clinical material.

A contemporary clinical example

The following material is taken from the supervision of a therapist who is an experienced clinical psychologist; he has not trained as a psychotherapist but has a wealth of clinical experience and a personality that inspires trust and respect in his patients.

> My colleague was working with a 50-year-old woman who had been the victim of sexual abuse by her father following her mother's death when she was 7 years old. The patient had led a difficult life, which had included a marriage to an emotionally

and physically abusive man. However, she had extricated herself from this, and after a number of other sadomasochistic relationships she came for therapy because she felt she needed help in consolidating a new relationship she had formed with a much more supportive man. The patient had had the insight that there was something in her that could ruin this new relationship unless she received help.

From what my colleague had gathered, the patient had been much closer to her father than to her mother, and prior to the mother's death they had enjoyed a good, non-abusive relationship. After his wife had died the father appeared to have suffered a breakdown and perhaps as a consequence the abuse had occurred. The therapy had reached a point at which the patient was exploring memories of having received emotional comfort and physical pleasure during the abusive activity. This was associated with her idea that she might have been ambivalent about her mother's survival, and she was beginning to consider the kind of oedipal issues that one would imagine in such a situation.

At this point the patient became extremely depressed, began to neglect herself badly, jeopardized her work and her new relationship, and spoke of a feeling that the sword she felt had been hanging over her for all of her life was about to drop. The therapist tried various interpretations, none of which improved the situation, and he became very worried about the patient. He resolved to change his approach and to talk to her about how she might cope better with her depression. He also said to her that he would discuss her case with her general practitioner and would suggest that she begin a course of antidepressants. However, the patient became more depressed and began to complain about the treatment and the awful situation it had brought her to. It was at this point that the therapist brought the case to supervision.

A dream was the central point of the session that the therapist presented in the supervision. The patient had dreamt that she was in a room from which she could see through a doorway into another adjoining room. She became a little anxious as the light in her room began to fade and eventually went out. She could still see because some light came from the neighbouring room. However, the dream became a nightmare as the light in that room faded, and she woke in an extremely anxious state as everything went black. She had one association: she attended evening classes in which participants tried to trace their family histories. She thought the teacher was excellent, but a difficulty had arisen: the caretaker of the school did not want the class to continue because it meant he had to work late, and he had started to turn off the lights before the allotted time. The teacher, a kind and gentle man according to the patient's portrayal (also an apt description of the therapist), seemed to be intimidated by this man, and the patient had tried to find ways of supporting the teacher by standing up for him.

As the therapist and I discussed this, we formulated the problem in the following terms: throughout her life, the patient had dealt with her guilt about the death of her mother and the subsequent abuse by the masochistic solution of colluding in the bad treatment of herself. She was now trying to break this pattern and live in a better relationship with her new friend. She knew, however, that her guilt would not let her do this and she had come for therapy to try to resolve this. As she reached that point in the therapy at which she had to consider what the causes of her guilt were (and also, of course, as she felt herself in the transference to be in a relationship in which she received relief and comfort), she had panicked. And, crucially, so had the therapist, to the extent that he had tried to work in a different way. The patient had understood this as evidence that her guilt was not able to be faced and had become extremely depressed.

I thought her dream symbolized this dilemma. The caretaker could be seen as a punitive superego who throughout her life had taken care to ensure that she was not happy. It now threatened her with the ultimate punishment—suicide—the lights going out before the allotted time. Her dream showed that she could bear this anxiety if the light in the neighbouring room stayed on. That is, if her therapist, the kind teacher who was helping her find out about her history, was not overwhelmed by anxiety and could in some way stand up to and shed light on the bullying and intimidating superego. All this she could dream, but when she sensed that the light next door had been extinguished and the teacher had been intimidated by the bully, no further thinking could occur and her capacity to dream broke down.

Discussion of the understanding given above formed one important part of the supervision session, and I used the material to teach the therapist about, for example, the superego and its pathological manifestations. However, I also spent a significant amount of time talking to the therapist about the emotional strain that the patient had imposed upon him. I introduced this into our supervision by saying something like: "This is a really good example of just how difficult it is—particularly, I think, when one is quite experienced and hence feels that one really does carry clinical responsibility—to deal with the unspoken threat that the patient might kill herself. I think in such a situation it is quite likely that we lose our faith in interpretation and try to find other means of helping the patient. But it is very important to try and resist this temptation and to keep trying to think what one's countertransference might mean. It's not easy, this is very difficult work emotionally." This led us on to talk about just how threatened he had been by this case, and he told me how he had come to dread her sessions and to imagine that he might be ill on the days that she was due. He also disclosed that he had had fantasies that he would hear that the patient had committed suicide and then of how he would be blamed by her family and shunned by his colleagues for being such an inept therapist. He had imagined that he would lose his professional reputation. This enabled us to elaborate how important it was to understand this very difficult countertransference as a communication about the patient's own superego and the way it had treated her throughout her life.

In the session following the above supervision, the therapist found an opportunity to say to the patient that she had really wanted him to understand how frightened she was if she thought about what had happened in her childhood, that she could feel so guilty she feared she could kill herself. He added

> that she had tried to get him to feel this fear in order to have it understood. In response to this, the patient said that she had been thinking increasingly about killing herself. Crucially, the therapist felt at that moment that this was told to him not as a threat but as a communication of an anxiety that the patient wanted him to understand. That is to say, the therapist had been restored as someone with a mind with whom she could communicate about her anxieties. Some capacity to think and consider had been regained. Her dream had detailed exactly at which point she felt she had lost this neighbouring, functioning mind, and it is interesting that it was exactly then that her capacity to dream had also broken down—she had woken up.

Of course this was not the end of the difficulties in this case, and we continued for the supervision of his work. Other difficulties arose, but the patient did eventually marry the new friend. Their relationship continued to be disturbed by her attempts to pull her husband into sadomasochistic ways of relating, but an increasing capacity to contain this inclination developed and she was more able to talk to her husband in order to enlist his help in stopping her attempts to ruin their marriage. Personally, I doubt whether one can hope for much better an outcome in such a case.

Discussion

In the introduction to this chapter I wrote that two benefits of a personal therapy were a greater tolerance of external reality and a greater acceptance of one's own thoughts and feelings, and I indicated the importance of these variables for a therapist's functioning.

It is extremely neccessary to help supervisees know just how damaged many of their patients are and what powerful anti-developmental forces govern their behaviour. There is frequently a strong resistance in the supervisees to knowing this. The aim of imparting such knowledge is not, of course, to destroy the therapists' optimism but to enable them to take a realistic view of the patient and to be aware of the limited progress the patient might make. Many patients have not had even the limited adequate parental care nor possess the perspicacity of the patient described above, and their prognosis is correspondingly poorer. A tolerant awareness of these grave limitations can *in itself* be a powerful container of the therapist's difficult countertransference feelings.

It is also vital to enable the therapist to be tolerant of the feelings that the patient invokes in him. In the example I gave, this included guilt of a persecutory nature and hence his thinking that he might be ill on the day of their appointment. (Usually the therapist hopes it is the patient who will be ill.) The guilt was linked to an overestimation of personal responsibility and associated resentment at being made to feel this. In addressing such phenomena, one must exercise tact; this must, I suggest, include never attempting to understand a countertransference difficulty in terms of the therapist's personal history or personality. I have found it helpful in such circumstances to use the pronoun "we", as in "It is quite likely in such circumstances we lose our faith in interpretation. . . ." This way of talking (I give it as an example of an attitude rather than a technique), as well as being an honest reflection of the fact that the supervisor knows from his own experience that such emotional strains are hard to bear, also communicates that one is talking about a professional difficulty inherent in the work and not a private, personal problem. Furthermore, describing a problem as one common to all of us helps the supervisee with his own difficulties about shame and the narcissistic vulnerability that exposing oneself in supervision entails. In this manner, some, albeit limited, modification of the intolerant superego that has been projected onto the supervisor can be made.

Very frequently, it is the patient who seems more aware of, and more disturbed by, the therapist's countertransference than is the therapist himself, at least as far as the patient can consciously articulate. This is the reason why it is of limited use to ask the therapist how he felt in the clinical situation: the answer is often not very revealing. The supervisor is much more likely to gain an insight into the dynamics of what is going on if he focuses on and analyses the *whole situation* rather than simply trying to understand the patient's pathology. One has to listen to the therapeutic dialogue as occurring between two people, *both* of whom are disturbed by what they have got themselves into.

An anxiety that might stop some practitioners offering supervision to untrained therapists is that it would involve them with people who are not serious enough about their professional development and who might even seek the status of doing psychoanalytic psychotherapy without putting in the hard work that this activity entails. From my experience, one recognizes such people in a relatively short period of time. Most notably, they have a great resistance to bringing process notes and undertaking close scrutiny of their clinical work. If one is prepared to take this up with them and, if necessary, terminate their supervision, then it is possible—although at the time unpleasant—to extricate oneself from a situation in which one feels one is colluding with something false or indeed even corrupt. This then frees one to make significant and important contributions to the work of those who are sincere in their wish to learn and to improve their clinical skills and who are working in situations in which such help can be invaluable.

This chapter is about the supervision of untrained therapists but I think its arguments illustrate the need for any therapist, no matter how experienced, to seek supervision or consultation at critical times. Whenever a patient's pathology is such that it goes beyond a therapist's capacity to understand, then there will be a temptation not to do the hard emotional work of working through the countertransference in a clinically informative way. At certain times this can lead to an impasse, and an outside opinion can then be invaluable in clarifying a therapist's blind spots. This knowledge of the perpetual struggle against the anti-developmental factors in one's own personality, and of the way that another mind can be used to help overcome them, allows one to approach supervision of untrained therapists with proper respect and empathy for their situation.

CHAPTER THREE

On the process of supervision in psychoanalytic psychotherapy

Montserrat Martínez del Pozo

Introduction

This chapter is based on the ideas of Freud, Klein, and other post-Kleinian authors—especially León Grinberg—and also originates from my personal experience of receiving and giving supervision. The supervisions have been carried out with psychotherapists in four-year training programmes in both the public and the private sectors (the Clinical Psychology Service of the Fundación Puigvert, Hospital de la Santa Cruz y San Pablo, Universidad Autónoma de Barcelona, and the School of Psychoanalytic Psychotherapy of the ACPP-AEPP). The clinical material comes from children, adolescents, and adults undergoing individual or group psychoanalytic therapeutic processes.

The relationship between the "learning position" and the different psychic positions in the supervision process and in the interaction between the various participants in the supervision unit

When a supervision process develops favourably, we become aware that we are submerged in a rich, complex, and shared process of evolution in which each of its components—the patient, the supervisee, the supervisor, the staff, and at times the institution—all experience a beneficial transformation. (In the 1970s, through a teaching programme, "Psychoanalytic Psychotherapy in the Public Institution", members of the Spanish Psychoanalytic Society—Bassols, Beá, Campo, Corominas, Eskelinen, Esteve, Feduchi, Folch, and Hernández—made it possible for systematic supervision to be inserted in the public-health network, contributing to a considerable transformation in the quality of service provision in mental health institutions.) We can then affirm, without a doubt, that skilled supervision is one of the most important channels for understanding the patient, as well as for transmitting and integrating theoretical, technical, nosographic, and developmental knowledge. Through a supervision we transmit knowledge to a therapist and a specific patient in a very live, personalized, sensitive, and thoughtful way, as well as know-how and a psychotherapeutic attitude actively based upon the emotional experience undergone in clinical practice. Also, supervision through a psychoanalytic psychotherapy framework allows a much broader view of emotional problems and illnesses, far beyond those of only the therapist–patient relationship.

Our aspiration is to foster a teaching and learning method much in the style of Bion, which implies a capacity for observation as well as participation, based on an emotional and intellectual commitment. The impact that this first experience exerts on the therapist is considerable and gives rise to defensive systems that depend on the conflicts evoked and the nature of the pain that these can entail. Over the years, I have been able to observe that although most psychotherapists overcome this crisis and evolve quite favourably, a few of them manifest personality disorders that hinder the patient's evolution as well as their own training.

In a supervision process, there are numerous factors that have a dynamic interrelationship, and these gives rise to multiple movements of progression and regression in each of the participants, who themselves oscillate in their unconscious use of the various positions—paranoid–schizoid, depressive, and sensorial (see Figure 3.1).

The *paranoid-schizoid* positions refers to a state of mind dominated by persecutory anxiety and in which the individual splits off and projects aspects of his self. This leads to states of mind such as emptiness and impoverishment, and also to paranoia as the object projected into will be experienced (through identification) as trying to project back unwanted aspects. Confusion of self and other will then be a common sequel. By the *depressive* position is meant a state of mind in which an individual experiences both loving and hating, cruel or destructive, feelings towards an object or objects. Guilt, concern, and reparative capacities are then possible or defended against by regression to the paranoid–schizoid position. By *sens-*

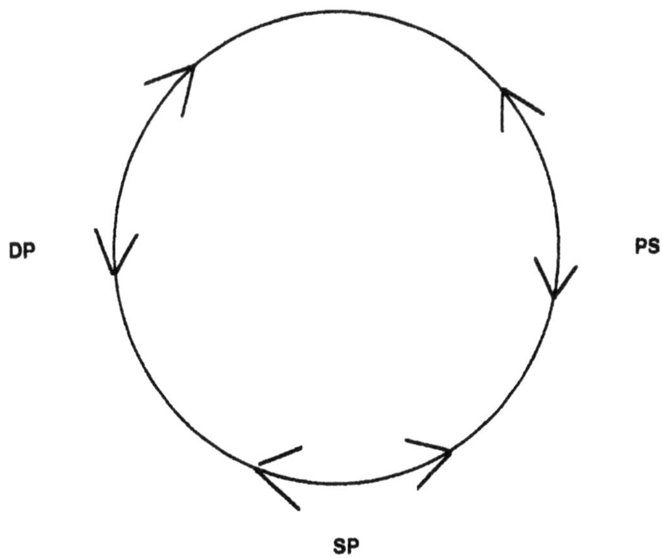

FIGURE 3.1 Diagrammatic relationship between the different positions (DP = depressive position, PS = paranoid–schizoid position, and SP = sensorial position).

orial position, I mean the maintenance of specific sensations to appease or recover from catastrophic anxieties, such as being shattered into fragments. The object in this situation is a "sensation-object" (Corominas, 1991). Ogden (1989) uses the terms autistic and autistic-contiguous. I use the term "sensorial position", as it is less specific in the pathology it implies.

An attitude that Dispaux (1994) calls "the learning position" emerges from the healthy dynamic interaction of these three positions. The essence of this concept lies in a true desire to study in depth not only theory and technique, but also the "soul" of the technique and of theoretical know-how. It is a question of being "touched", affected, altered by the supervision process.

In my view, the learning position is a personal attitude that predisposes one to think, to reflect upon feelings and emotions, and to feel the thoughts experienced in the psychotherapeutic relationship with the patient and with the supervisor as well as those belonging to oneself. These "feeling-thoughts" invite deep reflection about the patient and favour an integration of therapeutic know-how with therapeutic practice as well as with the therapist's own internal world, assisted by his own personal therapy. With experience, "feeling-thoughts" therefore become less defensive and stereotyped and increasingly personal and available for creative use. The learning position implies that the candidate has sufficient capacity and sensitivity to experience his own anxieties and defences instead of projecting them, and he is thus better able to understand himself and his patients. This attitude requires a capacity both to develop sufficient confidence in the supervisor and to differentiate self from objects.

The possibility of the learning position predominating in a stable way correlates with the capacity of the various participants to explore within themselves the oscillations between the various psychic positions so that a preponderance of the depressive position may emerge in the relationship with the patient and the supervisor.

In this chapter I consider the following aspects:

- the patient and his relationship with the therapist and the institution;

- the conditions and characteristics of the supervisor and the supervisee, including the relationship that the supervisor and the supervisee maintain with the supervisee's therapist (analyst or psychoanalytic psychotherapist);
- the relationship between supervisor and supervisee;
- the dynamics and characteristics of the staff;
- the characteristics and dynamics of the institution;
- the resulting combination of the various participants in the supervision unit. The individual transference and countertransference of each of these participants, in interaction with the transference and countertransference emergents of the group and institution, are of great importance (see Figure 3.2).

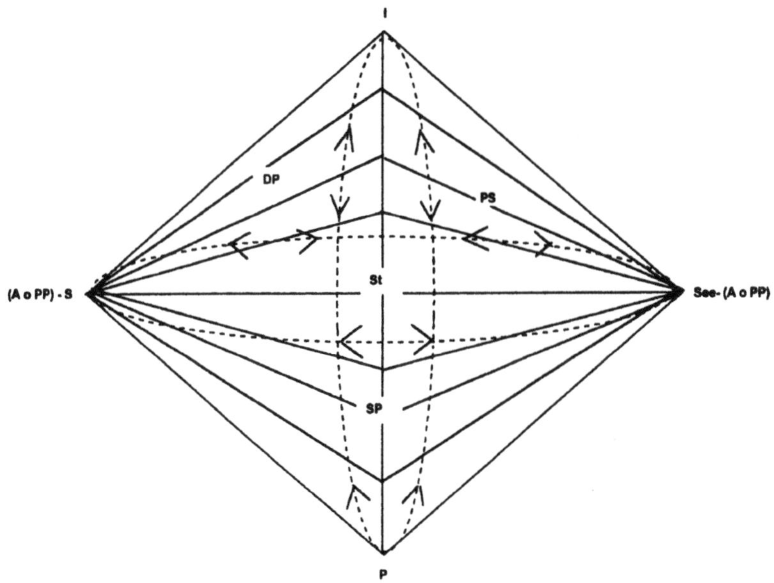

FIGURE 3.2 Diagrammatic representation of the dynamic interaction between the different positions and the participants in the supervision unit (I = institution; P = patient; DP = depressive position; PS = paranoid–schizoid position; SP = sensorial position; St = staff; S = Supervisor; See = Supervisee; A o PP = Analyst or psychoanalytic psychotherapist).

The supervision unit

The term that I use to describe the result of the interaction between all the participants listed above is the "supervision unit", which is based on the understanding that each individual has multiple aspects to his personality, and on an understanding of the dynamics of the group and its emergents (Folch & Esteve, 1992). The dynamic relationship between the various participants will be in a continuous movement between progression and regression, which will lead to a corresponding predominance of depressive position or paranoid–schizoid, or even catastrophic, phenomena.

These states or positions in an individual or group will have a greater or lesser effect on the patient's emotional life, but also on the other groups such as the supervisees and supervisor(s), as well as on staff relationships in the institution. In a similar way to family dynamics, supervision groups and staff groups in institutions are vulnerable to splitting processes, giving rise to subgroups into which progression or regression can be projected. These processes can evoke considerable pain for some of its members, which if regressive will interfere with their development or that of their patients.

EXAMPLE

The patient is a young man who comes for therapy on account of impotence and difficulty in ejaculating, and who also smokes extremely heavily. During the course of the sessions, he described the frequency and method of his masturbation and his dates with girls. In one of the sessions the patient reported that one of his aunts had become pregnant and had given up her baby daughter for adoption, which had greatly affected his mother. Recently, the therapist saw his patient as either very depressed or very hostile. In one session, the therapist felt confused, more so than usual in his work, and he also harboured considerable feelings of anger towards the patient. Throughout the session he was wondering whether to prescribe a pharmacological treatment for the patient's depression. Afterwards, the therapist tried to comfort himself by smoking a cigarette, his first after having given up smoking three months previously. He felt in urgent need of supervision and therefore asked one of his colleagues if he could take his turn on the rotation for supervision.

In his own treatment, he understood why this session had affected him so greatly when he recalled his own brother's marriage. He had made a girl pregnant and then married her, and recently they had divorced.

In the supervision, the therapist conducted a sincere and passionate defence of a pharmacological treatment, and on several occasions he wondered whether the supervisor's contributions were appropriate for his patient. Nevertheless, he went on with the therapy and brought a dream of the patient to the following supervision. It was possible from the dream to understand clearly the patient's struggle against identification with his uncle, an identification that, in one way or another, was related to his ejaculatory difficulties. At the same time, the therapist understood the way in which the patient provoked the therapist to identify and confuse himself with the patient. The therapist was able to understand that this problem was more problematic for him to deal with because of his own difficulties. This was also happening at a time when his wife was wanting them to have a second child, earlier than he would have liked.

This psychotherapy evolved favourably. The therapist was able to help his patient efficiently because he was able to come into contact (depressive position) with his own states of confusion and feelings of anger against the patient, which were blocking the treatment (paranoid–schizoid position). Through supervision, the therapist obtained insight into his own problem (depressive position) and was able to contain his acting out and trust the supervisor (depressive position and learning position). He was also able to get angry with the supervisor, doubt the latter's capacities, and project his own impotence and mistrust into him (paranoid–schizoid position), as well as temporarily fall back into his smoking habit (sensorial position), in order later to emerge once again in the depressive position and explore matters more deeply in his own treatment, in the supervision, and in the patient's treatment (depressive position).

The supervisor's perspective

When we initiate a supervision process, we try to transmit knowledge that emerges from our particular and idiosyncratic way of *combining* clinical experience, theoretical knowledge, and institutional possibilities. This triple confluence opens up an extensive and fertile field towards creativity.

Our purpose is to help towards an understanding of the patient, to outline the psychotherapeutic strategy, and to train psychotherapists. In addition to this, other objectives would be theoretical–technical and nosographic investigation, as well as research into the most appropriate learning systems for the training of psychoanalytically orientated psychotherapists.

In my daily experience over a period of twenty years, I have been able to verify that the kind of relationship established between the supervisor and the supervisee exerts an influence, in one way or another, on the relationship that the supervisee maintains with his patient and, consequently, on the understanding of the patient, on the psychotherapeutic strategy, and on the psychotherapist's training.

Relationship with the supervisee

Supervisors try to favour a relationship with the supervisee which is communicative and sincere enough so as to facilitate the patient's evolution and the psychotherapist's training. At the same time, we try to moderate the emerging anxieties evoked in supervisees in their work with patients so that they will be within limits that will allow for the feelings and phantasies that provoke the anxiety to be grasped consciously by the supervisee.

However, anxiety levels in the supervisor/supervisee relationship itself may become excessive if:

1. there are theoretical and/or technical differences between the supervisor and the analyst that are not conscious to the trainee;
2. the relationship that a young therapist and his supervisor maintain with the former's psychotherapist is such as to lead to a reactivation of primitive conflicts;
3. there are difficulties in the supervisor/supervisee relationship due to states or disorders, more or less temporary, in the supervisor and/or supervisee;
4. opposing interests—personal, scientific, professional, and so on—exist between the patient, supervisor, supervisee, staff, and institution;
5. there are institutional and staff problems that exert an influence on the supervision unit and, in particular, on the relationship with the supervisor, a relationship that is established initially as a result of the urge to know and investigate (Bion's K-link).

1. *Theoretical–technical differences between the supervisor and the supervisee's therapist*

In the first phase of training certain conflicts may arise from the theoretical–technical differences between the supervisor and the beginner's psychotherapist. If their perspectives are very different, this can provoke states of great helplessness and disorientation on the part of the supervisee, who feels misunderstood and at times rejected by the supervisor. It requires a great capacity as a therapist to treat one's first case with only the support of what one understands in the supervision, without the aid of what one understands from one's own treatment. At the other extreme, an excessively similar orientation can establish a "honeymoon" type of relationship with a certain tinge of collusion, which does not promote new thought processes. In my view, in the supervision of the first case, there should be a coinciding theoretical base. However, I would also point out that different nuances and variations in the particular approaches can also foster greater depth in one's own treatment and in the patient–supervisee–supervisor relationship.

2. *The relationship that therapist and supervisor maintain with the former's psychotherapist and reactivation of primitive conflicts in the supervisor–supervisee link*

The supervisor nourishes the supervisee with his clinical, technical, and psychotherapeutic know-how. However, he also carries the responsibility of assessing the supervisee's capacities and progress as a therapist. This intensifies the supervisee's anxieties as to whether he will be allowed or denied the possibility of becoming a qualified psychotherapist. Depending on the vicissitudes of the supervisor/supervisee relationship, especially in the supervision of a therapist's first case, there can be a reactivation of primitive conflicts in the supervisee which can make him feel that his survival as a therapist is threatened.

It is important to bear in mind that the nature of the conscious and unconscious, real and phantasied, link between the supervisee's therapist, the supervisee, and the supervisor will influence the supervision process.

In the unconscious mind of the supervisee, the figure of the supervisor is deeply associated with that of the parents. Parents, in the history of the Greeks, had a right over their offspring's life or death. Aeschylus, Euripides, and Sophocles have personified these primitive conflicts of survival and the tragic repercussions that they entailed:

- The King of Thebes' *fear of being murdered* by his own son leads to the abandoning of Oedipus-child in the mountain so that he can be devoured by wild animals, and Oedipus-adolescent, in his "lack of knowledge," *kills* his father at a crossing. Jocasta, his mother, does not recognize her son in her husband's absence and loves him too much. Oedipus, *blinded by his love for his mother and his greed for power,* marries Jocasta and is crowned King of Thebes. Ridden by unconscious guilt he ends up investigating and pursuing on the outside what he cannot investigate inside him. When Oedipus withdraws his projections and connects with "the truth", it becomes so profoundly unbearable that the tragedy is unchained.
- Clytemnestra *kills* her husband in order to *avenge her daughter's sacrifice,* her loneliness, and her jealousy and arouses her son

Orestes' anger, who then *avenges his murdered father by killing his mother and his stepfather.*

- The father replaced by the brother in Antigone unchains all kinds of wars and *provokes aggression towards the tutor* who dares take his place.

Olivier (1995, p. 8) raises the following questions concerning the father, which I would extend to both parents and to the process of supervision: "Is it possible for one not to feel unconsciously resentful towards that parent who ignores or despises in his son or daughter that part of himself which he has begotten and raised?" I would ask whether it is possible for one not to feel resentful towards a supervisor who is too distanced from the work that the analyst or psychotherapist is carrying out with the trainee therapist, or who discredits—be it verbally or through his attitude—the professional practice of other supervisors respected by the student. What occurs when, through identification, it is the subject himself who identifies with that parent and despises one of his parents inside himself, thus attacking his internal objects? How can you get out of this zone of confusion and obscurity, in which one does not know where projection and projective identification finish and the parents' primitive conflicts begin?

In my opinion, such processes can be found to be active in the first processes of supervision. Young therapists have been in treatment for only a short time and are not usually fully aware of how these conflicts affect them, and without their realizing it they run the risk of reproducing them through processes of identification with their patients. For this reason, it would be of great interest to establish a supervision of supervisions.

3. *Psychopathological tendencies in both supervisor and supervisee*

The supervisor's psychopathological tendencies can alter the process of supervision, interfering with the understanding of the patient and the evolution of the trainee therapist. These disorders can be aggravated as a result of their peculiar combination with the supervisee's own pathology. For example, depressive states in a supervisor may lead him to not recommend psychotherapy to appropriate patients who consult him (especially if the supervisor's experience is more of psychoanalysis than psychotherapy); manic states incite pseudo-maturity in the therapist as well as in the patient; narcissistic states promote the disqualification of other colleagues; paranoid tendencies lead to a distrust of the therapist's contributions; and so on.

4. *Opposing interests*

The supervisor's blind spots in his own analysis—excessive and fanatic adherence to a psychoanalytic theory; an intense desire to supervise a specific institution, staff, or person; excessive preference for one of the staff members; an interest in treating or not treating particular cases; or conflicts in function of one's theoretical or personal motivation—all inevitably lead to disturbances in the supervision process, in the staff, and even in the institution.

5. *Institutional and staff problems that influence the supervision unit*

However, beyond the psychopathological tendencies in the supervisor, one must also point out the oedipal difficulties that at times emerge within the staff. These tendencies arise not only on the part of the supervisees but also on that of the supervisor and the management of the institution. If the two latter functions happen to coincide in the same person, the dynamics of the supervision can be influenced depending on the post the supervisor occupies in the hierarchical scale of the institution and the relationship that the participants maintain with the different supervisors. On occasions, depending on certain dynamics of the supervision group, evolution and progress is projected into some of its members, whereas regression is deposited into others.

If the supervisor colludes with these defensive systems, this can generate considerable disturbances not only in the supervision process and in the patient, but also in the professional relationship among the members of the staff. In my opinion, there exists a two-way oscillation between the transference and countertransference of the supervisor, staff, and institution and the supervisee and patient (whether individual or group).

Given the repercussion that the dynamics of the supervision unit exerts on the therapeutic groups, it is very important to ensure group cohesion in the staff.

EXAMPLE OF GROUP SUPERVISION

In a supervision it was noticed that the two supervisee group co-therapists, when presenting group analytic session material, tended to establish dual relationships with the supervisor—one tended to use a seductive technique, the other used sincere appraisals accompanied by a competent manner; one tended to masochistic submission, the other to idealization—and the group as a whole tended to use one of its members as a scapegoat. The co-therapists commented on a group session in which, to a certain extent, the following aspects could also be observed: rivalry with the more active therapist, the formation of subgroups of two, and the choice of a scapegoat. Enriching associations were given by different staff members. The supervisor picked up on these, developing and connecting one contribution with another, thus favouring dialogue and thought and working-through of her own group countertransference towards this particular group of patients and therapists. She stressed those contributions that she considered the most useful, making an attempt to discourage those that arise from the seductive, masochistic, etc. areas, and of course including contributions made by the group member used as a scapegoat, thus stimulating introspection and the genesis of meaning. Subsequently, she made a synthesis of the emerging dialogue, including the various alternative hypotheses, making an attempt to avoid the creation of subgroups of two and the appearance of a scapegoat in the supervision unit. The ongoing working-through of conflicts in the supervisees' personal therapy group as well as supervisions that favour group cohesion improved the supervisees' work with their own patient group.

Understanding of the patient: observation and the technique of listening

One fundamental aspect of the supervision is to provide the supervisee with a good-enough understanding of the patient. In order to accomplish this it is absolutely essential *to foster the art of observation and listening*: to observe and listen without projecting one's own conflicts into the patient, without invading him intrusively with one's own wishes or theories, "without memory and without desire". This is a tremendously complex and difficult task, for which reason it is of the utmost importance to reflect upon the supervisee's interventions, observing the dynamic interaction established with the patient, and analysing the transference and countertransference.

Catharsis

As far as catharsis is concerned, we will never be able to emphasize strongly enough how positive its effects are. For this reason, during the supervision it is convenient for the supervisee to perceive the beneficial effects of sincerely transmitting the difficulties experienced with the patient, as well as those that may be experienced in the containing function that the supervision provides. This experience in the supervisor–supervisee relationship will favour the expression of the patient's painful feelings and their possibility of being contained by the psychotherapist.

Coherence in the theoretical model

I would stress the importance of keeping coherence in the theoretical model; such coherence can facilitate the refutation of hypotheses and theories (Popper, 1972) and at the same time favour a dialectical attitude, which McDougall (Ithier, 1984) calls "floating theorization". This consists of maintaining an attitude in which theories give shape to the clinical material but without invading it intrusively. The observed material, which includes the interaction between the patient and the psychotherapist, can strongly reverberate with our theories and lead to their modification (Coderch, 1995).

The search for therapeutic strategies

In institutions a basic objective is to promote the search for appropriate therapeutic strategies through research on focal treatments, group techniques, family and couple therapy techniques, and so forth, bearing in mind a triple confluence:

1. the patients' characteristics;
2. the trainee's level of experience;
3. the potentials of the staff and institution.

The therapist in supervision

During the process of the first supervision, different stages can be observed: the initial impact, the relevant moments of enthusiasm, of decreasing interest, of crisis, of calm, of termination, and so forth.

The initial stage

Psychotherapists are receptive to the projections and projective identifications of their patients, which gives rise to states of disturbance and emotional vulnerability, which in turn interact with their own personal conflicts and lead them to seek psychological treatment. This state of vulnerability is much more pronounced in the trainee therapist who has not yet undergone enough time of personal psychotherapy and lacks sufficient theoretical–technical support. For this reason the trainee therapist will need, more than ever, to be contained and helped to work through the countertransference by the supervisor, who will help to discriminate between the psychic states and emotions that derive from the patients' projections and those that derive from the therapist.

EXAMPLE

After having given an account of the case, and despite the fact that the patient has provided sufficient material, we experience difficulty in being able to associate. We have the feeling that there is something that separates us from the patient, who is perceived as being distant. The therapist comments that she often experiences this feeling and that she thinks it is due to her own personal difficulties and lack of training. She feels empathy for the patient but when she is with her, without quite knowing why, she often feels sorrow. Perhaps she doesn't understand her! She feels sorrow but at the same time experiences a feeling of lack of contact. The supervision proceeds in the same atmosphere . . . and we come to the agreement not to rush too fast in trying to understand. We consider that it is necessary for the therapist and the patient to deepen their relationship. Simultaneously, we support the therapist by manifesting that, in our view, her lack of understanding is not a consequence of her lack of training. Two months later, in a session close to the summer holidays, the patient mentions a slight pain in her groin and then proceeds to associate this with a conversation held with her mother in which the mother commented that the patient had been hospitalized for three weeks as a result of a complication after an operation for an inguinal hernia. When the therapist asked her how old she had been then, the patient answered, "three months", and after a silence she explained with great emotion that while she had been hospitalized her mother would look at her through the glass window, crying, and couldn't help thinking: "You're so seriously ill, and I can't take you in my arms and comfort you!" This understanding of the countertransference related to this biographical information led to considerable insight in the psychotherapist as well as in the patient.

During this stage, the trainee becomes intensely aware of his own lack of knowledge and of the knowledge that others possess, which activates strong feelings of dependence on the supervisor as well as fear of his critical judgement. However, I have observed, as Rosenfeld did (Ithier, 1984), that the therapist in whom the learning position predominates is generally willing to expose what he did and did not do, as well as his feelings and emotions regarding the patient. This attitude implies that the supervisee must have a self with a good-enough capacity to sustain himself in the fluctuations between "integration–disintegration". In the initial period this aptitude is put to the test since the trainee experiences the supervision not only as a place where he can become aware of the patient's difficulties but also of his own, thus acquiring greater insight into his personal internal conflicts. The therapist's intuitive awareness that there exists the danger of confusing himself with the patient arouses intense fears and doubts about himself, about his own psychopathology, and leads him to wonder whether he has what is needed to practice this profession. Therefore, the process of supervision not only becomes a place where he can relieve himself of doubts regarding the patient, but also constitutes a process in which multiple questions are raised about his own personal and professional capacity. The evolution of his training will depend on his capacity to sustain himself at moments of crisis and on the extent to which he is capable of keeping the ability to feel and think about the patients.

In the beginning, any proposal made by the patient—a change of time, questions of a personal kind, holiday breaks, prolonged silences, interviews with the parents, and so on—generates considerable anxiety in the supervisee. And the transference? "What is the transference? Why do I not grasp it? What is wrong with me?"

Awareness of one's lack of knowledge, doubts about oneself, the emotional turmoil of this initial stage, and so on can lead the supervisee to omit his interventions and participate little in the supervision; to project his many doubts and insecurities into the patients; to cling rigidly to norms or theories; to idealize the supervisor (which, if very extreme, can generate adhesive identifications that inhibit the capacity to learn from his own experience and develop his own thinking); or to soothe his insecurity by looking for a hasty institutional promotion. At the other extreme, we can also observe a tendency to oppose any form of setting or norm and to pursue a defensive heterodoxy.

Intermediate stage

In the intermediate stage, the therapist finds himself more confident and a certain stage of stability is inaugurated in which he feels freer and more capable of deepening the emotional experience with his patient, laboriously thinking about it in private. As a result, learning is reinforced and this is a good time to supervise with different masters and contrast different theoretical–technical contributions and perspectives. This incipient security can also inaugurate a certain healthy competition and rivalry with the supervisors.

The final stage

In the final stage of our four-year training process, an evaluation of the learning process is usually carried out, and the therapist anticipates a sense of loss, which leads to a strengthening of the processes of introjection. However, in most psychotherapists one can observe a certain acting-out resulting from the confluence of mourning for the ending of their patients' psychotherapies with mourning for the ending of their own training process.

The best way to contain these anxieties is to facilitate thought processes and the generation of meaning by promoting the evolutionary aspects of each individual in the staff, simultaneously favouring the processes of "differentiation–individuation" as well as those that promote group cohesion. At the same time, the tension derived from the perpetual individual–group conflict must be kept within acceptable boundaries. In this way an atmosphere capable of generating insight is favoured, which is re-invested in the group creativity, thus facilitating mutual benefit for the individual as well as for the group.

States of disturbance or disorders derived fundamentally from the supervisee's personality

On some very few occasions, when confronted with the anxiety that the practice of psychotherapy and supervision entails, I have experienced how some students fall back on radical defences. In these cases I have observed a predominance of omniscience and a direct application of theoretical knowledge. These same therapists can become rivalrous with their supervisors, discrediting the latter's "poor" theoretical training while idealizing other supervisors. Others, after an experience of intense emotional participation, distance themselves from the patients and have serious difficulties maintaining the *internal setting*. The more paranoid ones experience the supervisor as someone who can threaten their professional development, and so on. If such difficulties become chronic, their roots must be analysed thoroughly and the appropriateness of going on with the supervision must be assessed.

Institutional supervision

In some circumstances, the staff members find themselves trapped in certain institutional conflicts which then infiltrate the patient's material and the dynamics of the staff and the supervision. We must not forget that the unconscious and its defensive systems exist in institutions and can become organized in such a way as to attack permanently the possibility of individual and social transformation. They can become deeply rooted in the different levels of the staff, who can then remain in permanent collusion, defending against dynamics that could generate creativity and change. However, some institutions are able to develop forces that can redress the balance of destructive and/or regressive aspects. Institutional supervision is one of these forces. It favours communication and awareness of one's own destructiveness, and the possibility to contain it; it allows a clarification of roles, and it keeps in mind not only how long the therapists have been in training, but also how long the staff and the institution as a whole have been in training. All this helps to discriminate those feelings that emerge from dealing regularly with patients manifesting specific characteristics from those that derive from the organization's pathological defences.

Clinical and institutional supervision can contribute to working through the pain that results from individual and social limitations and can mitigate the envious attacks that arise on account of the creative and intimate relationship of therapists with patients.

The aspiration to interpret "without memory and without desire" is essential in the process of supervision. It is true that through this attitude we are less likely to avoid working through pain, but this precisely is when psychotherapists foster their humanity—in the light of their being finite, in the ethics of their limits and tolerance of "not knowing". It is by recognizing one's own grief as well as that of others' that hope and joy are generated. Vitality and reason, nature and culture, emerge from the awareness of the limitations of human knowledge.

Synthesis

In the supervision process the following must be considered:

1. the manifest and latent motivation of each of the participants in the supervision unit;
2. the psychopathology and foremost conflicts of each of the members of the supervision unit and of the unit as a whole;
3. the principal ways the patient, each member of the supervision unit, and the whole together "teach and learn";
4. the relationship between the supervisor, the supervisee, and the latter's therapist;
5. the need for the supervisee to be in an advanced stage of his treatment;
6. neutrality on behalf of the supervisor;
7. a certain theoretical affinity in the first years;
8. the supervisor's experience in dealing with groups;
9. respect for the setting;
10. the need to establish a supervision of supervisions in certain situations;
11. the incorporation of new members into the supervision unit by consensus;
12. the time dedicated to each of the cases as a function of various interests;

13. the socioeconomic situation;
14. the supervision unit constitutes the group emergent, in which the conflicts and capacities of each member are projected and wherein the Oedipus myth and its relation to knowledge acquires particular importance for its understanding.

CHAPTER FOUR

Supervision in mental health teams and institutions

Ulrich Streeck

Introduction

Psychic and social factors exercise a lasting influence on the manifestation, progress, and treatment of mental diseases. In addition to pharmacological and social therapeutic treatment, psychotherapeutic means can positively influence psychotic disorders. Furthermore, the relationship to the patient of the therapists involved in the treatment, the relationship of the members of the therapeutic team to one another, and the institutional conditions in general, all play an important role in the progress of the disease and its treatment. Experience of this has led to an awareness of the importance of recognizing and understanding these psychosocial conditions, with their diverse and complex relationships in psychiatric institutions, in order to create the requirements necessary to influence them therapeutically. Supervision is designed to achieve this goal.

Attitudes towards supervision

Attitudes towards supervision in psychiatric institutions have long been conflicting, and one still occasionally meets with reservations and ambivalence. The majority of therapeutic co-workers regard supervision as indispensable, but sometimes one also encounters the viewpoint that supervision in psychiatry—particularly psychodynamically and psychoanalytically oriented supervision—is superfluous or even harmful. Unrealistically high expectations are occasionally attached to supervision, but supervision is also at times regarded as a luxury that is contrary to the essence of psychiatry. Sometimes the prospect of supervision awakens anxiety because it is associated with control and surveillance. Such fears are especially strong in institutions that operate, as do many psychiatric hospitals, in the force field between therapy and state control—though again, false hopes may be attached to supervision as a means of liberation and self-government. With the prospect of supervision also arise fears of a subversive element that could endanger the familiar security and routine of day-to-day psychiatry, while, on the other hand, supervision may become the focus of illusory hopes for relief from untenable situations.

For the most part, one encounters hopeful expectation and fears simultaneously: desire for support and rescue on the one hand, and scepticism and fear of control, exposure, and intrusive surveillance on the other (Salvendy, 1993). Furthermore, a predominantly biologically oriented psychiatry has seen a renaissance over the last ten years; under its influence, a noticeable tendency is reemerging in some places to neglect unconscious aspects of communication and the dynamics of therapeutic relationships in psychiatric institutions and to attribute little importance to these with regard to diagnostic and therapeutic questions.

The roles of supervision

Supervision is not a clearly defined method. There are various types of supervision, depending, for example, on theoretical and clinical orientation, but also on the subject area that occupies the foreground of supervision, or depending on different aims and methods. Despite differences in emphasis and detail, supervisors in psychiatric institutions should have a competent understanding of interpersonal relationships, especially of how interaction and communication in didactic and multi-person relationships are influenced by the unconscious and by transference as an expression of conflictual, internalized object relations. In their interpersonal relationships, psychotic patients in particular employ, among other things, non-verbal means of interaction, the effect of which is difficult to escape for those dealing with them (Gabbard, 1992; Roughton, 1993). Communicated through unconscious ways and means, enactments (Johan, 1992) develop between patient and therapeutic staff which cause patient and therapists to behave like figures from their own pasts (projective identification). The patient not only then experiences the therapist he is speaking to as if he were some earlier person (transference), but this therapist does indeed himself behave like the person from whom the patient is transferring. This is known as countertransference enactment (Gabbard, 1995).

Such processes of unconscious communication and interaction can be exposed and examined through supervision (Fleming & Benedek, 1966). In this way, a deeper understanding can be reached as to the complex interpersonal relationships between patients and therapeutic personnel, and new approaches towards a changed relationship can be explored.

Before a psychiatric facility invites supervision, or a supervisor takes on an assignment, a clear understanding should be reached as to the subject area under scrutiny, what the objective is, and the kind of supervision required. The more clear and unequivocal this is in the beginning, the more likely unrealistic expectations, which lead to unnecessary disappointment, can be avoided. Within psychodynamically oriented supervision, there are various possible focal points. Perhaps it is the working relationship between members of the institution amongst each other that occupies the foreground, or perhaps the professional working relationships within a team. On the other hand, however, interest may be focused on the medical treatment by therapeutic personnel and—impossible to consider separately—on the relationships between therapeutic workers and their patients. The first type of supervision includes consulting at institution level and team supervision, which is primarily oriented towards the working relationships of therapeutic co-workers. The second type focuses on case-oriented individual, group, and team supervision, as well as on Balint group work (discussed later in the chapter). Though these distinctions are hardly ever strictly observed in practice—in the real day-to-day supervision of psychiatric institutions, team- and case-oriented supervision, for example, usually flow into one another—it is still useful if client and supervisor agree in advance as to the objectives towards which the supervision is aimed.

Supervision of teams and their working relationships

In psychiatric institutions, the treatment of patients is not usually the responsibility of a single doctor or therapist, but is the task of a treatment team in which members of different professional groups cooperate. The dynamics of the relationship between the team members is closely tied to the psychic and interpersonal disturbance of the patients for whose treatment they are responsible (Tucker et al., 1992). The pathology of the patient can be reflected in the relationships of the therapy staff. For example, polarized conflicts between subgroups within the team can reflect the divisive defense of patients with borderline personality disorders (Kernberg, 1984). In a reverse manner, however, conflicts between team members can also affect the psychopathology and the interpersonal relationships of individual patients and relationships within the patient group—aside from the poor effect such conflicts have on the professional efficiency of the team itself. With the help of team supervision, the unconscious dynamics of these relationships and each team member's share in relationship events can be recognized and examined. The main focus of supervision may lie more strongly either on the working relationship of the team members to each other or on the relationship of the therapy staff to the patients. *Personal* relationships between team members should not be the object of supervision in the institution. There is danger, where this is not observed, of the team supervision being extended into an encounter group, the usual result of this being that the working relationship within the team is disturbed even more seriously than might have been the case without supervision.

The aim of the type of team supervision that focuses primarily on the working relationships among therapy team members is to determine whether the cooperation, assignment of responsibilities, decisions, and spheres of authority agreed upon by the team, with a view to their common task, can be effectively understood and implemented. Team supervision with this focus therefore concentrates on areas where it is important to discover and understand the conscious and unconscious obstacles to cooperation and communication in the team that stand in the way of effectively accomplishing their task and assists individual team members to participate in this task. When successful, supervision helps a team to maintain or recover its professional efficiency.

The main prerequisite for the type of team supervision that focuses on a team's working relationships is that the therapeutic treatment of psychiatrically disturbed patients is indeed organized as team work. A number of staff with various professional qualifications who work with one another does not yet constitute a team. Sometimes therapeutic workers who speak of team work have only the vaguest idea of the form of their cooperation. Their work and their functions are not organized as a team. On the contrary, this is a weakly structured group in which distinctions of authority, competence, responsibility, or decision-making power are blurred or even denied. In a team, on the other hand, the division of labour is efficiently organized; workers have clear roles and functions; qualifications, experience, and degrees of competence are taken into account; and responsibility, authority, and power are divided amongst different members of the team.

Another important requirement for team supervision that has the aim of improving working relationships is to establish as clear an idea of aims and tasks as possible through the teamwork model. This model should illustrate who does what in the team, with whom, and towards what end for the patient. Without such a model, there is the above-mentioned danger of supervision diffusing into a self-exploratory event, which in turn will have a destructive effect on cooperation within the group of therapy staff. In some cases, a supervision with the aim of improving a team's working relationships can help a group by finding a model of another, cooperating team for them to observe and learn from.

Without doubt, the self-exploratory needs of workers in psychiatric institutions are justified and deserve to be taken seriously. However, they should not be treated within the scope of supervision. Team supervision is also not the place to deal with a team's cooperation and communication problems if these do not emanate from within the therapist group itself but arise from the objective institutional conditions under which the team works. Problems resulting from the hierarchical division of power and decision-making in the general institution are as unlikely to be solved within the scope of team supervision as problems resulting from an individual's lack of competence.

Supervision of the team's therapeutic relationships with patients

In the type of team supervision most often carried out in psychiatric institutions, the relationships between the therapy team and the patients play a central role. Here, too, the team should be in working order, with well-defined tasks and functions and a clear division of responsibilities. If this is the case, supervision can become a forum where important areas of unconscious relationships, dynamics, and the psychopathology of the patients are examined and understood.

In psychiatric institutions, the therapeutic staff often work under considerable stress to act and respond quickly. Supervision gives them a space where this pressure is lifted and in which they can reflect on the tension and urgent impulses that come from their often severely disturbed patients, without their having to react to these immediately. Given adequate framework conditions for the supervision, workers are not directly exposed to the chaotic, aggressive, and sometimes shameless or harassing behaviour of the patients. In the supervision situation, they can obtain adequate inner distance and examine and understand the patient's behaviour and their own response to it in a space of reflection. This leads to a deeper understanding of the patient's inner world and of his pathological relationship behaviour, and it opens up new approaches for dealing therapeutically with these (Adelson, 1995).

Patients with psychotic disturbances or severe personality disorders tend to violent acting out. In working with them, it can easily happen that a line is overstepped. Autonomy and dependence, interpersonal nearness and distance are fraught with grave conflicts. As a result of structural deficits, they lack the ego-functions necessary to deal adequately with these existential demands (Blanck & Blanck, 1974). In team supervision, problems that are related to the overstepping of boundaries are often raised. Dealing with such serious disturbances requires stable and reliable framework conditions. They are an important condition for maintaining good and reliable therapeutic relationships that are neither too close nor too distant. This framework is indispensable for the treatment of such patients. For many patients, the therapeutic process represents a way along the framework (Kernberg, 1973), and it may actually turn into a struggle for the framework itself. The framework provides support and orientation, guarantees reliability, and keeps boundaries intact. Supervision often becomes a central place in which the overstepping of boundaries is recognized and where, through mutual effort, framework conditions are re-established.

Serious problems can also arise when different members of the therapeutic team have different experiences with the same patient which appear to be at variance. Each team member may have a different view of the patient. At first sight, these different pictures might appear to have nothing in common, as if the therapists were not even looking at the same person. This is usually the effect of a fragmentation by psychotic patients or of massive splitting defense mechanisms. This can easily lead to fierce conflict between members of the team, with each team member representing a different non-integrated side of the patient. Team supervision provides an opportunity to bring together these various sides and fragments, thus contributing to a more whole, integrated picture of the patient. Views of the patient that were different for each team member can be recognized as various partial aspects, which are ultimately seen as belonging together. This in turn can lead towards the first steps in a patient´s integration.

Occasionally, guidance, instruction, and the transference of competence from experienced colleagues to less experienced ones in a psychiatric institution is called supervision. However, the goal here is neither to improve or maintain the efficiency of a therapy team nor to discover and examine unconscious conflicts and fantasies related to transference and countertransference processes. Predominant in such instances are the activities of guiding, directing, conveying information, and advising. Hence, they should not be described as supervision.

Balint group work

Balint groups were originally developed by Michael Balint as research seminars to study psychological implications in general medical practice. The seminars revealed that "the most frequently used drug in general practice was the doctor himself". The study moved on to examining the "pharmacology" of the doctor as a drug, its form, frequency, curative and maintenance doses, hazards and allergies, and so on as revealed in the doctor–patient relationship (Balint, 1964, pp. 1–5). Such groups have also proved useful for examining the relationships in psychiatric institutions between professional staff and patients.

Since their beginning, Balint group methods have developed into a valued instrument for further training. Balint groups have long ceased to be carried out just with doctors in family and private practice, as was originally the case, but now include clinic doctors, medical students, as well as members of other professions such as social workers, theologians, and teachers.

In a Balint group, which usually contains eight to ten participants, a member will report spontaneously on his experiences with a patient or client. From this develops a discussion in the group on the relationship between the reporter of the situation to his patient or client. It is one of the tasks of the Balint group leader to examine, with the help of observations, ideas, and support from the group, the implications of transference and countertransference and to make clear to the doctor, nurse, or social worker in question how this unconscious behaviour affects a particular relationship. According to Balint, the aim of this group work is to help doctors to become more aware of what is going on, consciously or unconsciously, in the psyche of the patient when doctor and patient are together. When a Balint group achieves this:

> the acquisition of psychotherapeutic skill does not consist only of learning something new: it inevitably also entails a limited, though considerable, change in the doctor's personality. [Balint, 1964, p. 299]

With the aid of Balint group work (according to his formulated aim), a helper should be placed in a position to recognize his own emotional reactions—even if they shame him, even if he despises the reactions, even if he tends to condemn himself for them—so as to be able to adjust these emotional reactions to the patient's illness. Instead of reacting to the unrecognized emotions that underlie his relationship with the patient, he arrives at a deeper understanding of his patient, which in turn allows him to find fresh approaches to therapeutic treatment.

The Balint method belongs to applied psychoanalysis. With the help of this method, unconscious areas of a relationship may be examined and understood in order to change them if necessary. With regard to its use in the field of clinical psychology, an occasional objection is heard that unconscious relationship elements in professional staff and psychiatrically disturbed patients are irrelevant to the understanding of severe psychiatric illness, or are at least of marginal importance. This is usually not so much a statement of scientific knowledge of psychiatric—especially psychotic—syndromes than a rationalized emotional devaluation of the patient.

Balint group work cannot be a substitute for further training of personnel in psychotherapy. However, it is a goal of Balint group work to recognize the emotional aspects of relationships in both patients and staff that hinder full professional involvement and effectiveness in psychiatric activities.

Consulting at an institutional level

Consulting in institutions for psychiatric care can be efficient and helpful in cases where changes affecting the institute as a whole are planned and undertaken, and where, therefore, the entire social network of the institution is involved. In order to help solve basic communication and cooperation problems in the organization—for example, between different departments or between administration and medical and/or therapy spheres—it can be useful to bring in a supervisor from outside as an institutional consultant.

Problems affecting the institution as a whole are often a result of organizational difficulties, and often of leadership problems. Supervision at institution level is aimed at examining unconscious determining factors in the interaction problems of an institution. It is not designed to help solve fundamental organizational or administrative problems. In such cases, it would be more sensible to seek advice from an organization consultant with training in sociology rather than from supervisors trained in psychoanalysis.

Consulting to an institution is applied social science. In Germany, unlike in the United States or Scandinavian countries, it is a poorly developed speciality—especially in the field of psychoanalysis—and in less demand than other types of supervision and consulting. One reason for this is that social services and their bureaucracies, which also includes psychiatric hospitals, are usually organized along the lines of classic administrative bureaucracies: that is, the client has no significant influence on the type and scope of service or the organization of work (Fürstenau, 1978). Such conditions offer little motivation to make any change in traditional structures or the way work is organized.

The psychiatric hospital is a social organization in which members of different professions must work together in mutual dependence at close quarters and in an extremely complex social and communication network. It is highly sensitive to disturbance but is also particularly sluggish and resistant to institutional change. There are, therefore, a number of potential areas for the application of institutional consultation which can help detect and relieve basic underlying cooperation difficulties that impede effective work. Institutional consultation can also offer support when new basic therapy methods are to be introduced into psychiatric institutions, if such methods involve a new distribution of responsibility, power, and decision-making among members of different professions—for example, if the principle of a therapeutic community is to be introduced.

Institutional prerequisites for supervision in psychiatric hospitals

Whoever conducts supervision and Balint groups in institutions for psychiatric care should be familiar to some extent with the conditions in the institution.

The supply of staff, both of doctors and nursing attendants, is insufficient in some psychiatric institutions. In many institutions, nurses and doctors would often be overtaxed if they became emotionally engaged with each patient. Sometimes, too, the fluctuation in staff is quite high in psychiatric clinics, particularly with regard to nurses, because of part-time and shift work, so that there is little constancy in the relationship between professional helpers and psychiatric patients. Although it would be sensible from a therapeutic standpoint, and often more than necessary, it is almost impossible to assign to a seriously disturbed patient his own permanent nurse. Sometimes, due to difficult institutional framework conditions, the responsibility for patients is unclear and fragmented, especially when members of different professions participate simultaneously in the treatment of a patient and each person's sphere of responsibility has not been specifically agreed on beforehand. The therapeutic sphere is especially handicapped and impaired if there is interference from administration in the therapeutic sector—for example, with regard to staff planning, the assignment of beds, or the length of a patient's stay.

Reliable and sufficient institutional framework conditions are important prerequisites for stable and reliable cooperation and undisturbed communication among the professional staff, and for a satisfactory relationship between them and the patients with whom they are entrusted. Occasionally, however, it may be observed that difficulties in cooperation and communication within the team are rationalized with the argument that the institutional conditions are unsatisfactory, when the reason for the problem lies elsewhere, namely in the relationships within the therapy team. Consistent, sufficiently long-term, and supportive emotional relationships require supportive institutional framework conditions. Unfavourable conditions have a negative effect on cooperative working relationships, especially on the relationship between therapy personnel and patients. The consequence of inconsistent, non-supportive institutional conditions can easily be that therapeutic relationships remain shallow and not meaningful, or that the behaviour of therapy staff becomes restricted to a more or less pragmatic treatment of patients. Such an emotional distancing of staff from the patient is supplemented by the tendency to describe the psychiatric illness of the patient in exclusively descriptive psychopathological terms, and so thus to view it—as Balint says—as a single-person psychology. This enables them to ignore the possibility of a two-person psychology—that is, the *reciprocal* relationship between professional staff and psychiatrically ill person.

If the supervisor is unfamiliar with the framework conditions of a particular psychiatric institution, he will not be in a position to estimate adequately the influence of these conditions on the emotional relationships in the psychiatric ward, and he is unable to judge accurately the reasons for any possible disturbance of, or hindrance to, relationships.

Stable framework conditions are also important for the implementation of the supervision itself. They are an important condition if supervision is to be used as a setting in which participants can speak freely and express opinions independent of the institution. The more reliable the framework conditions for supervision are, the greater is the likelihood that an atmosphere of trust can develop, one in which participants can work with one another without anxiety in a mutual effort towards understanding.

The framework conditions required for supervision include a clear arrangement as to the regular time, frequency, and duration of meetings, the place of supervision, discretion concerning confidential communications, and the composition of the participating group. Irregular participation and sporadic absences cause a high fluctuation in the composition of the supervision group, whereby resistances against the supervision often arise. The more unclear the framework conditions arranged between supervisor and participants, the more likely such resistances are to develop. These are also displayed by participants leaving the supervision group too early or arriving late—often with the pressure of duty as an excuse.

Finally, a clear agreement as to what the supervision will involve is most important. Thus, for example, it should be established whether the working relationship of the team members among themselves is to be the focus of the supervision, or whether this should be the team–patient relationship. Usually both areas are discussed at the same time, but this too should be a matter of consensus before the supervisor begins his work. Last, but not least, the supervisor should arrange with the participants that a topic of discussion should be agreed upon at the beginning of each session, on which they should then express themselves as candidly as possible (a basic rule).

Professional staff in clinical psychiatry are constantly subjected to severe emotional strain in their work. The daily contact with psychiatrically ill patients often awakens violent emotions, conflicts, and fantasies. Driven by necessity, staff protect themselves with the aid of intrapsychic, psychosocial, and institutional defences and conformity mechanisms. The practised, habitual, and professionally accepted role behaviour of colleagues in psychiatric hospitals, which also fulfils psychosocial protective and defensive functions, contributes to this further. Supervision can offer helpful support here by assisting workers in psychiatric care to become aware of unnoticed, unconscious elements in their treatment and in their relationships to one another and to the patients entrusted to them, thus enabling them to employ their full professional and personal competence for the benefit of severely mentally ill people.

CHAPTER FIVE

Supervision in a hospice for AIDS patients

Peter-Christian Miest

The setting

The care of terminally ill patients confronts caregivers with a set of specific stresses and requires effective institutional support such as regular supervision of the staff.

As Vachon has recently pointed out in her comprehensive review (Vachon, 1995), this necessity has received much attention by the modern hospice movement. This chapter reflects some of my experiences over the past five years of supervising carers in a nursing home for AIDS patients. Prior to the supervision there had been an alarmingly high turnover of personnel; it was hoped that, through supervision as a form of caring for the caregivers, this turnover could be reduced.

The supervised institution is a twelve-bed hospice with about thirty-five, mostly part-time, staff members chosen from diverse occupational fields. The hospice admits patients who, because of their AIDS illness, have in some way come to need additional care. They therefore exhibit all kinds of features of terminal bodily breakdown. It can be that a patient, because of a psycho-organic brain condition, needs not so much physical care but rather a cognitively and socially supportive environment; or that a patient, who until now was cared for by relatives, takes advantage of the infrastructure of the hospice and moves in—even with his relatives. In exceptional cases, and when there are beds available, patients who suffer from a terminal illness not caused by AIDS will also be admitted. Not all patients who come into the hospice die there. After all, it is typical with AIDS that totally unanticipated deterioration or improvement in the condition occurs. This sometimes leads to patients being able to return to their previous surroundings after a phase of intensive care. Frequently, they are readmitted after a few months, when their condition again worsens. The composition of the group of a maximum of twelve patients changes rapidly and randomly, depending on which patients were just admitted and which have already left or died. The mean length of stay of a patient in the hospice is forty-five days. From the nature of HIV infection it will be readily understood that intravenously injecting addicts and homosexual men are the most frequent patients.

In the beginning

The first question that occurred to me was, how could this large and constantly shifting team—at that time thirty-five people, changing on a daily basis—be supervised in a meaningful way?

I made the following suggestion: the team would be divided into three groups, and every two weeks I would meet with each group, outside the hospice location, for discussions about their work. Through this suggestion, I tried to interrupt the ceaseless rotating caretaking action by incorporating spaces in-between, so as to create for the staff a setting for quiet reflection. As a psychoanalytically thinking supervisor, all I could provide at this point was to make time available and, within that time, to offer a friendly, non–action-orientated climate that would encourage the staff to pay evenly suspended attention to all uttered comments.

Next to the omnipresence of death as an external reality, a world of inner realities should come to exist—a world of feelings, thoughts, fantasies—or, in short, a world of symbolic meanings. The frighteningly rapid succession of deaths that seemed to drown out almost all other needs, thoughts, or feelings had pushed the team into ceaseless frantic action. No sooner had one of the patients died, and any attached feelings of grief barely formed, than all the attention had to be turned immediately towards the next intensely needy patient. Often it seemed as though the staff's own limits with regard to their ability to withstand stress had no consideration. A member of the team suddenly broke out crying during one supervision session, but within a moment she took a tissue and was almost apologetic and smiling again, "I'm OK now . . ."

Time for mourning

Not by chance does time play a central role in the mourning rituals of our culture. Traditionally, black mourning clothes were worn for a full year; church memorial services took place a month after death; remarriage after being widowed was only allowed after an appropriate time. Many cultural elements point to how much the process of mourning requires time. If this mourning process is interrupted too soon, or is layered over by one or even several more losses, the work of mourning will be incomplete—the remaining emotions must be suppressed and will then express themselves as symptoms. In the situation presented here, these emotions were in part grossly resisted depressive feelings, which often manifested themselves in chirpy upbeat bantering or in repeatedly resurfacing states of total exhaustion.

The team now integrated into their work routines two concrete aspects that proved to be very helpful.

The first was the introduction of a mourning ritual, in which the staff retreat for a few hours every eight to ten months to remember together the many who had died in the previous period. Understandably, sometimes the name of a patient has already disappeared from memory; sometimes the visual image of the patient can no longer be recalled. Here it helps to have in the office a constantly visible board with the names and photos of former patients on it.

The second ritual was the setting up of a small room as a "room of silence". Staff, patients, or even relatives can withdraw to this when they need protection from disturbances. The room is comfortably, but also somewhat monastically, furnished and is entered with a certain respect—almost like a room for religious worship.

* * *

The establishment of the supervision setting created a protected space for reflection. Psychological realities could now begin to withstand the repetitive onslaught of death. After the supervision setting had been strengthened by the two additional measures that I have just mentioned, we could then begin to process together the diverse psychological features that came to light.

Summarized below are three of these features. The first refers to death, especially the issues of parting, separation, and remaining behind; the second refers to dying and matters of holding and repulsion by the psychological as well as the physical disintegration; the third is AIDS itself as a cause of death, and how the themes of addiction and sexuality run throughout work with AIDS patients.

Death and survivor guilt

At the moment of its appearance, death divides people into the dead and the surviving, and although this very division is perhaps the most temporary and deceptive one we know, in the case of a specific death it cannot be questioned. Furthermore, when we consider the narcissistic tendency of all the helping professions to split between "sick and healthy," between "needy and without any needs", there is for those who work with the dying a further intensification. The split then becomes "mortal" versus "immortal". I had the impression that this split was sustained by both sides—that is, by the patients as well as by the staff. "*And what do* you *know about unbearable pain*?" might be one such reproach from a patient to his care-giver. And on the side of the staff there were countless situations where they tried to make the impossible possible, as if their basic helplessness, actually their mortality, should not come to light. Even in the supervision sessions themselves we saw this split mirrored—for example, when I was told that I had no clue about the work in the nursing home, *"You sitting so comfortably in your analyst's practice"*. I became aware—more than once—how much I tried to cover up my not-knowing in the face of some of the situations discussed in the supervision, replacing it with a seeming all-knowing. Just as, in the face of death, the split between "dead" and "living" always guarantees the survival of the living, so I also felt a distinct reluctance towards one member of staff's suggestion that I should defer my role as supervisor for a week and instead work with them in the hospice as a care-giver. Then I would "Know what it is we're talking about in the supervision". I must have feared not surviving as the supervisor—that I would in some way "be pulled into death"—and turned the offer down, though not without feelings of guilt.

As I became aware of my own guilt feelings, I asked myself if there might not be a parallel guilt feeling in the staff members towards their patients. At first this could not be made conscious until I had repeatedly shared the following observation: I expressed to the team that I always got the impression that there reigned in the hospice a climate of very special warmth, and that the dealings of the supervision participants with one another were—especially in the moments of greeting—of an almost compulsive loving attention. I carefully posed the question as to whether this peculiarity of the team, this climate of loving interaction, could also be understood as a defence mechanism. My caution seemed necessary to me, because I could not totally rule out my own envy of the undoubtedly gratifying closeness of the team members with one another. After a time of being gently persistent, I was successful in uncovering the defence. It became clear that the team had put up an almost impenetrable shield of thoughtfulness, tenderness, and loving attention to protect themselves from the always active spring of survivor guilt. The guilt of the survivor in the face of the dying is a psychological phenomenon that has come to our attention through research into traumatic situations. Primarily through work with victims of the Nazi concentration camps, but also through work with the victims of natural disasters, accidents, and violent crimes, we know that this specific and generally very burdensome feeling of guilt can arise whenever the traumatic event does not hurt all victims equally. The less traumatized, the less seriously injured, or the surviving victims seem to be forced by the power of the trauma into an identification with the perpetrators or with cruel fate. In the case of carers for AIDS patients, this survivor guilt arises in the helpers as a powerful psychological phenomenon. We are all at the mercy of this still incurable disease; we are all potential victims, and yet today we are "by chance" standing at the bed of a dying person. "By chance" I mean that there is really no just reason why he should die and not I. And if we consider now that a large portion of the hospice staff themselves come from the high-risk group of homosexual men, and some have already lost friends or even partners to AIDS—and if we consider that even among the heterosexual staff members it was frequently the loss of a close acquaintance or even partner that was the deciding motivating factor that led to working in the hospice—then it is no longer surprising how much the feeling of "sitting in the same boat" and having to watch as one after another falls overboard can produce immense survivor guilt.

Unconscious aggression

It is well known that where guilt feelings exist, aggression is not far off. In the preceding section I defined survivor guilt as an unconscious identification with the aggressor and thereby implied that the aggressive affect does not have its origin primarily in the helper but only secondarily—from his identification with the aggressor or, alternatively, the terrible catastrophe. I believe, though, that the guilt feelings, which were able to be recognized more and more clearly in the supervision sessions, did not spring only from the guilt of surviving. It seemed that, throughout, there were also guilt feelings related to genuine aggressive affects of the staff towards their patients. For example, when a patient who had grown close to the hearts of the whole staff group, because he had shown himself over the course of time to be a very considerate and grateful patient, requested three days before his death to be transferred to a general hospital and then actually died there (without the individualized trusted company that he would have been guaranteed in the hospice), there was, mixed in with the confusion and lack of understanding, a significant amount of anger towards the patient, who had so abruptly disavowed, snubbed, and abandoned the team. Here I must add that a large part of the staff's motivation to work in this hospice developed from disenchantment with previous posts in traditional hospitals. So one could easily empathize with the staff's feelings of being snubbed—the very wish to die in the traditional hospital where conditions for dying are so inviting of criticism seemed downright absurd in the minds of the staff.

However, it was not only this transfer that called forth the staff's anger; I heard just as clearly that they felt especially cheated out of the death of this patient, as it would surely have been a beautiful, moving, and conciliatory death, where there would have been, for once, some small compensation for so many wretched, degrading deaths. I think that, on the one hand, the injustice of this patient gave the team the opportunity to reveal aggressive affect, but that, on the other, the cause of this emotion lay deeper. The fact of death itself has always carried the distinguishing characteristics of abandonment and will thus inevitably trigger aggression. Recall the findings described in Bowlby's attachment theory (Bowlby, 1980): an experience of separation produces first the aggressive feelings of protest, then feelings of resignation or, in the case of a successful grieving process, sorrowful affects. We understood in the supervision that the team was exposed not only to a repetitive and constant overlayering of fresh feelings of grief, but also to a repetitive surfacing of feelings of aggression which, though generally unconscious, were no less decisively present in their daily work. Here I think the supervision takes on an especially important preventive function, as we know that, especially in the areas of care for the seriously ill, the danger of aggressive handling of the patient is not minimal. Again and again we are confronted with frightening news of the murder of ill patients which are presented by the perpetrators as compassionate acts of mercy, behind which, however, is enormous unconscious aggression. How close they are to such catastrophically aggressive outbreaks is often barely acknowledged by nursing teams. This makes it even more urgent that there is a continual working through of this set of problems and feelings.

That we succeeded in this was thanks to a persistent difficulty the team had with a patient who suffered from Amyotrophic Lateral Sclerosis (ALS) and who was totally paralysed with the exception of her face muscles and was dependent on the staff for every task. She was no longer even capable of speech. When originally admitted, she was categorized as terminal. However, this was several years back. Her condition, described upon admission as a terminal state, continued to deteriorate as her paralysis extended to ever more important life functions. She was truly not an easy-to-please patient. For example, when she was put to bed for the night she would signal again and again with her eyes that the pillow under her head was still not positioned right. She focused on every fold in the pillow, and her despairing demands that the staff should do more for her became ever stronger: they should spend more time with her, they should focus more sensitively on her needs, they should not take any days off, because someone new would then have to start again with the sensitive search for the right positioning of the pillow. In summary, the care of this woman, dependent to the highest degree on the help of others, became a relentless fight for constant attention without any limits. In this, the team felt forced to spend excessive amounts of time in every act of care for her. The smoking of a cigarette and the drinking of a glass of water would require more than an hour. One staff member after another was worn down by this battle and sometimes quit explicitly because of her: a few times it was stated, "either she goes or I do". It took countless supervision hours with the most heated eruptions of rage and powerlessness before a tolerable balance of claims to professional care, on the one side, and the need for limits to such demands, on the other, could be found. The patient continued to live, against all expectations. It became very clear that the great strength of this team, with its quick, uncomplicated, and highly empathic ability to react to new and unfamiliar situations, was mainly with short-term patients. Their capacities with this patient, however, repeatedly threatened to fail. She survived year after year, seeming also to "survive" many members of staff. In the ever-more unbearable tension between her demands and the capabilities of the staff, death surely would have been a relief for the team—maybe also for the patient. What is this thought, if it is not a death wish? Such a deeply disturbing realization was necessary, yet so painful, for all. Where death had taken over as a merciful outcome for all the other patients, bringing at some point an end to their suffering and thereby also ending the powerlessness of the staff, and where death had "acted" before the staff could develop a death wish towards the patient, it refused this service in the case of this patient.

AIDS

Whereas, in the previous section, thoughts about grief, guilt, aggression, and death appeared as rather abstract phenomena, the following aspects focus on the actual process of dying. Consider the AIDS illness: a virus slowly and progressively destroys the immune mechanisms of the body, rendering it vulnerable to a multitude of infections that will eventually kill the person. The type of secondary infection can differ greatly, as can the course of the illness. Skin changes such as Kaposi's sarcoma with its typical black spots and open wounds that will not heal often appear, as do fungal infections with widespread areas of peeling skin. Often this external disfigurement of the body is made even more apparent by significant weight loss. In the meantime, an extremely unpleasant odour can develop to which neither the patient nor the caregivers can adapt. Infections in the brain can destroy individual motor, sensory, and cognitive-psychological functions, leading to diverse convulsive syndromes, psycho-organic psychosis, or full-blown dementia. All of these processes can occur rapidly and without warning, can alternate, or can combine. If you try to imagine all of this, and add to it the always present danger of staff becoming infected themselves with the deadly virus, you will surely understand why every member of staff is asked again and again: "*And you can stand this*?" One understands then also why there are so many part-time employees in the hospice, and why such attention is paid to making sure that the amount and duration of the least tolerable strains must have limits. The staff members are indeed exposed to extraordinary pressures: after all, they strive to fulfil the therapeutic plan of the hospice, which is to give the patients holistic, loving care, to offer the often poorly socially integrated patients a "holding environment". Therefore, in no time at all, they often get into intense relationships with the patients, which sometimes cannot be clearly differentiated from those that would be appropriate of relatives.

Physical holding naturally plays a central role with respect to care of the body. The patients must often be physically assisted, which is not possible without intensive body contact. If, on the one side, dying, with its unstoppable erosion of the patient's energy, brings the patient down into a bedridden state eventually pulling him into the grave, so, on the other side, do the caregivers prop up the patient, right him again, and brace themselves against his dying. This physically imagined power is directed as much against the patients'dying as it is against the caregivers' own disgust and physical revulsion at the bodily disfigurement. As with the notion of aggression, we also encountered in the supervision a considerable resistance to taking notice of the idea of disgust. I understood this not only as a fear of not being able to live up to the ideal of the dispassionate, attentive nurse; I suspected much more, that as the disgust became conscious, the intrepid fight for life would take on a threateningly ambivalent character. I was vehemently corrected by the team members every time I spoke of "the house of the dying"; it was "a house of the living!" I understood that where disgust causes the holding to become brittle, the direction of physical attention can suddenly reverse, so that what was holding can become a letting-fall or even a pushing-away.

In conclusion I would like to sketch out a thought that relates to the psychological meaning of the main routes of becoming infected with AIDS. I refer to the sexual as well as the addiction aspects. Both sexuality and addiction were originally—that is, in the infantile context—forbidden areas and were reserved for the parental figures. Violating this ban would lead to real punishment, and also, on a symbolic level, there was the threat of punishment by castration. When in our adult lives we encounter a person with AIDS, we are faced with an anachronistic phenomenon, as though the infantile fantasy that sexuality and pleasure would lead to death has become real: this patient seems actually to have been sentenced to death for his sexuality or his addiction, as we once feared—and we thought that the fear had been long since overcome. Depending on the maturity we ourselves have reached in the realms of pleasure and sexuality, we may be confronted with feelings of ambivalence, disgust, seduction, and desire. These manifestations were developmentally appropriate in our childhood and adolescence. Today, however, in the context of adult-helper and patient, these reactivated emotions cannot unfold without conflict. So, for example, revived infantile curiosity can creep into the daily work with patients as an inappropriate sexualizing, which then tends to be rationalized as an occupationally necessary interest. One staff member recently commented, very sarcastically, that she would like to know how close to the anus of a patient a near-sighted (homosexual) colleague would have to draw his face to be able to accurately assess his decubitus ulcer. This question was aimed directly into the highly frightening connection between the sexuality of the patients and their illnesses and their deaths and the sexuality of the staff members. Archaic fears lie in wait here, and the question as to whether the team supervision will allow these issues to be worked through remains an open one.

CHAPTER SIX

From action to thought: supervising mental health workers with forensic patients

Dorothy Lloyd-Owen

Introduction

The Portman Clinic is a national resource, an out-patient clinic within the public sector, offering psychoanalytic psychotherapy to children, adolescents, and adults, who come with problems of sexual perversion, violence, or delinquency. It is a small clinic, staffed entirely by psychoanalysts and psychoanalytic psychotherapists, some of whom are psychiatrists, others having backgrounds in psychology, social work, or related disciplines. Our understanding of our patient group is based firmly in clinical practice and developed through research and training.

Consultation and supervision are offered to colleagues in primary forensic settings, such as special hospitals, prisons, regional secure units, and the probation service. The vast majority have no psychoanalytic background, and their approach is, broadly speaking, behavioural and cognitive. Ostensibly, these colleagues come to the Portman Clinic because they want to learn and think more about the psychodynamic approach to understanding their patients/clients and their task. However, in my experience they actually come because they feel themselves to be impoverished or frozen, and they find that their one-dimensional techniques leave them ill-equipped to deal with forensic patients who are highly disturbed. Such a sense of impotence means that they often come for supervision with the expectation (and hope!) of being offered a magical solution.

I supervise these colleagues individually and in small and large groups. Although not psychoanalytically trained, they seem to come with the classical Freudian subdivision of the psyche into id, ego, and superego clearly in their minds. They describe their patients as if they had well-structured egos which occasionally struggle in conflict with the forces of the id, and they view their own interventions as equivalent to engaging a superego (themselves) in the battle. This assumption has complex effects on their relationship with me. Their contacts with their patients tend automatically to take on a paranoid–schizoid character in which everything is experienced as a threat and where people are related to, not as whole people but in terms of an aspect of them that has a function. Part-object relating, splitting, projective identification, idealization, and concrete thinking abound. They often initially view me in one of two ways: either as a persecuting superego whose influence is perceived as threatening and potentially destructive or, if non-challenging, as that of the id.

EXAMPLE

A social worker pays a home visit to a female client suspected of child abuse and drug abuse. Looking in through a window, she notices a man giving himself an intravenous drug fix. When the client opens the door, she is clearly under the influence of drugs and her child is running around out of control. The worker confronts the woman about her drug-taking, which she denies. An impasse ensues and the social worker leaves, worried, furious, and feeling helpless. The client, without doubt, felt both attacked and abandoned. The supervisor, too, is in a difficult position—either she is seen as attacking the social worker's approach or, if she tries to focus on and understand the dynamics, she risks being perceived as presenting no challenge.

The patient–worker couple

In a sense, it is a *couple* that is brought to supervision. One part of the couple is the perverse and/or delinquent patient, often poorly motivated for treatment, and who frequently resorts to action in order to communicate and evacuate what is internally unbearable. The other part of the couple is the worker, generally lacking understanding of unconscious processes and unaware of transference and countertransference issues.

The worker tends to relate to the patient at a concrete level, focusing on the acting-out as if an intellectual understanding on the patient's part will lead to altered behaviour. In this kind of scenario, a mutually persecuting relationship often develops. The patient may also gain a sense of the worker's basic good intentions through his efforts to help, feeling that there is some appreciation of his (typically) traumatic history. Ambivalence thus pervades the relationship.

Most patients in forensic settings possess an early history characterized by poor or abusive object relationships and attachments. This early experience of an ambivalent, non-comprehending object is frequently re-enacted in the patient–worker relationship. Such re-enactment in the transference, while expected in psychoanalytic work, is often unavailable for understanding in primary forensic settings. The situation becomes further compounded by the public nature and expectations of the worker's role: the legislative system and public opinion accord an omnipotent role to the agency and hence to its workers. As the worker's omnipotence inevitably gives way in practice, however, to helplessness and a sense of persecution, these feelings cannot be processed within the agency and end up being re-projected into and located in the patient. Such diversely opposed feelings—omnipotence and impotence—are also true of society's approach to forensic agencies, where the expectation of magical "cure" swiftly becomes denigration of any skill when patients enact their conflicts in the public arena.

The supervisor as persecuting superego

It is at the beginning of the supervision process that the supervisor may be experienced as a persecuting superego, destroying this familiar paranoid–schizoid functioning of the couple and offering no immediate replacement.

The following example demonstrates typical features of this kind of interaction.

EXAMPLE

The worker was responsible for the supervision of a patient who had caused considerable raised anxiety through his alleged stalking of a well-known female pop star. The patient saw the star's manager (also female) as the "devil" and wanted to warn the star against her. It was known that this man had felt compelled to leave his birthplace, where his sister remained in his mother's care. All professionals who had had any contact with this man found themselves terrified. Exploration in supervision revealed no evidence he had ever harmed or attempted to harm anyone. Nevertheless, anxiety predominated in the worker and her agency, and thinking could not take place. The man was clearly very paranoid, if not suffering from a formal psychiatric illness. It seemed clear to me that the worker and her agency were experiencing in the countertransference the client's terror of his own internal conflict in relation to a "managerial" mother, and that this inhibited thinking in both client and agency. The pressure of this process was such that the agency managers reacted in a persecuting way to the worker, crudely examining her records and interrogating her to establish whether or not she was doing enough to stop this man's stalking, despite her very able management of the case. The worker was then made to feel even more uncontained, terrified, and helpless. Yet she was drawn to action, involving other agencies, to assess and protect his family, as if he were in danger of abusing them. I suggested that she arrange a psychiatric assessment for her client and inform him of this. In doing this, the terror left her and became manifest in him. She was able to think again and in particular to think about her counter-transference. She then began to appreciate that her patient's aim had been to protect his sister/himself/his family against an immensely powerful evil mother-figure in the way he wished to protect the pop star against the evil manager. This shift enabled him to be properly understood as being ill and hence to receive in-patient treatment. The worker found that she recovered from her disabling state of anxiety and terror that she would be killed.

The importance of the environment

Through my supervision of these colleagues in the forensic field, it has also become very clear to me that many of their settings are uncontaining and seem to function as paranoid–schizoid institutions. In Britain, this has been significantly exacerbated by a government that treated people as part-objects in a money-driven culture, as described by Bell in his paper, "Primitive Mind of State" (Bell, 1996). Bell examines the introduction of the "market" into the National Health Service, viewing it from the perspective of the destruction of the Welfare consensus. He suggests that the ideology of the "market" and the attack on "welfare-ism" derive considerable support from the fact that they appeal to primitive parts of the personality, parts that view dependency or vulnerability as weakness—a process originally described by Rosenfeld, who termed it "destructive narcissism" (Rosenfeld, 1971). Bell also suggests that the NHS reforms create fragmentation and alienation. He postulates that this has led to primitive survivalism which, although a natural outcome of the process described, will prove very costly in terms of its effects on morale—an essential component in adequate health-care delivery. This primitive state of mind is an institutional defence against the anxiety of not being able to meet well-demonstrated and previously understood needs in worker and patient groups, a phenomenon described in detail by Menzies-Lyth (1960). At the government level, it seems that envious attack predominates and good whole-object–based practice has to be denigrated. In the NHS, the present reality is that patients are referred to as "products" and can receive treatment only if funding can be arranged with their local health authority. Agency survival is the primary task, pending a change in current government policy or the economy.

The probation service in England and Wales has the statutory responsibility for managing the majority of perverse and delinquent members of society. The fundamental ethos of care and control has recently been redefined (not internally but from outside, by the responsible government department) and limited to only control. Astoundingly, the traditional requirement of a social work training, which at least embraced some dynamic casework values, as the basic preparation for work as a probation officer, has been eliminated by government, and pressure is being put on a demoralized probation service simply to confront symptoms. The client can no longer be treated as a whole person. Furthermore, cuts in funding and the threat of job losses have produced an enforced acquiescence within the service. The resultant ethos is that of the claustrum, as described by Donald Meltzer, with its identificatory and claustrophobic consequences (Meltzer, 1992). This phenomenology of projective identification with internal objects, according to Meltzer, is twofold. Its identificatory aspects are generally recognized as grandiosity, hypochondriasis, and depressive or confusional states. The projective aspects are rooted in the splitting processes (of the objects and of the ego) and are manifested as perversions, addictions, and paranoia in which the person feels incarcerated. Perverse patients undoubtedly evacuate their claustrophobic anxieties into their therapists. Where the therapist also finds himself in the prison of a perversely denigrating institution that demands that he intrude into the patient with the aim of omnipotent control, the therapist's claustrum seems complete. Perhaps reassuringly, some staff in these settings continue to struggle to relate to patients as whole objects/people against a pressure to process them cost-effectively as part objects. This often leads to them feeling overwhelmed by the ill and damaging nature of their patients, who often project their sense of guilt and responsibility into the workers; the latter, in the countertransference, feel blamed and lose sight of the patient as a whole.

The supervision process and the "depressive position"

The workers who come to the Portman Clinic for supervision enact and contain the parts of their institutional systems that are in touch with a wish for a more healthy "depressive position" way of being (Klein, 1935). However, the very process of psychodynamic supervision, which encourages the worker to think about the client as a whole person whose behaviour can be seen to contain symbolic meaning, generates in the worker pain characteristic of the depressive position. This (as we all know) is hard to bear and can lead to a state where the supervisor and the supervisor's clinic is idealized or envied until eventually internalized. When the pain can be borne by the worker, he or she may be attacked through envy by his agency when he begins to put understanding into practice. In becoming independent of the institutional defences, the worker is seen as rocking the boat, threatening the homeostasis, and he then becomes vulnerable to attack by his envious and anxious colleagues.

EXAMPLE

I was asked to supervise a specialist team who worked with long-term prisoners in the category of the highest risk to society. I was initially given a one-year contract, renewed for a second year. It emerged in the supervision sessions that these workers felt at times overwhelmed and nauseated by the prisoners' offences, which included murder, serious sadistic sexual assaults, rapes, and other forms of extreme violence. Their agency's expectation was that they should do something with these prisoners to make them safe upon release.

There was also the problem of the institutional defence of the prison, which essentially utilized splitting. Each prisoner was seemingly related to and regarded by prison staff as either "cured" or "incurable"—either end of a spectrum, with no view of any intermediate, more complex position. One consequence was that prisoners would be moved from one institution to another in a way that reflected this blunt categorization. The team often saw through this, as a result coming into conflict with the prison staff. Between them, the two groups re-enacted the internal world of the offender, who reduced his objects to split "cured/good" or "uncured/bad" ones. For example, when early release on parole was being considered, this could be supported by the prison staff on the basis that the prisoner had responded to, say, a cognitively based anger-management programme, and opposed by the visiting team-worker who could observe no real change in the prisoner's capacity to relate to objects. The prison staff could be viewed as good by prisoners—and indeed agreed with by them—since they had an investment in their treatment programme. The visiting worker would be viewed as bad by both prisoner and prison staff, and splitting became paramount. Supervision allowed this re-enactment to be thought about. Having the whole team present for supervision was invaluable: they unilaterally re-enacted the split between worker and institution and then allowed it to be thought about as belonging to the prisoners' way of defending against thinking and feeling. This, in turn, informed their practice, and they redefined their task as that of undertaking an ongoing pre-release risk assessment based on their understanding of the prisoners' object relationships. In a subsequent routine Home Office (the government department responsible for prisons) inspection of the team, their work was acknowledged to be of a high standard. Then financial restrictions led to the news that this specialist unit was to be closed and the work transferred to other workers, who did not want it. This policy decision, based purely on finance, was one where contact with prisoners was to be reduced to a frequency prescribed by a formula rather than need. The workers were informed that they faced possible redundancies. However, they were told that the contract for their supervision at the clinic for the remaining period of the second year could continue.

This attack on them and their work, and on me, was hard to bear. In the absence of a containing management structure they had no validation of their work and their depression gave way to annihilation anxiety (one of the earliest, most primitive anxieties and one often experienced by their damaged patient population) in relation to their own work and future. They had once been the depository for patients that no-one else wanted, and they were identified with those patients in their colleagues' minds: denigrated, feared, and therefore unsupported. They were also envied for their capacity to think about and work with these prisoners—to survive, as it were, and to think about the conscious and unconscious processes at play in the drama in the manner described by Bollas (1992, p. 207). My function was then to hold in mind their value both as professionals and as human beings. The needs of their patients as well as society also had to be contained, so that the workers did not give up. It was as if for a time I had to become more of a therapist than a supervisor (as these were workers without therapists) until they could survive what they experienced as an annihilatory attack, and one which was compounded by them in their identifying temporarily with their aggressors. They needed help to think about ways of validating their work, if only by writing it up so that it might enhance the understanding of those who were (unwillingly) to succeed them. Equally important was the need for the workers to negotiate for themselves new positions that reflected their skills, albeit that these skills—which had caused breaches in the agency defences—might again work against them.

There existed for this group of workers a tension between their understanding of their patients' illness and dangerousness, and how this might be addressed within an agency that had had, as a defensive manoeuvre, to evacuate such understanding. (This process is described as a reversal of alpha functioning, in ridding the psyche of thoughts, by Bion, 1962, pp. 25, 101.) They also had to avoid polarization: that is, the pressure either to comply or to continue to be perceived as a danger, which would have to be concretely controlled or itself be evacuated from the agency. At the time of the "attack" on these workers I was more than ever acutely aware they were not in analysis and lacked the individual therapy which might help each with the internal meaning of these events and their impact. Equally they did not have an internalized theoretical framework, as would an analytically trained worker. There was thus considerable pressure on the supervisor to make sense of what was happening rather than get caught up in it.

The supervisor and the process

In thinking about this supervision process, important considerations must be given to timing, pace, and degree of input and drawing out. The supervisor becomes invested with the whole "package" and therefore has to be aware of his own narcissism as well as of the risks of idealization and, later, denigration (since the supervisor ultimately will not fail to disappoint). If the supervisor does not recognize these features in the countertransference, there is a likelihood that projections will be re-projected unmodified.

Yet arrangements for regular, at least weekly, supervision are often resisted, perhaps couched in terms of funding and workload or that, somehow, fortnightly supervision is seen as more tolerable. This may reflect, amongst other things, core complex anxiety where desire for attachment, fear of engulfment, attack and flight, and the further sense of emptiness and need of attachment pursue each other in circular fashion (Glasser, 1992). Dependency is resisted in the dis-service of need.

EXAMPLE

Some four years ago I was invited to sell myself, in competition with a behavioural supervisor, to the staff group of a residential unit offering assessment and treatment of families known to have abused their children. The choice between the two quite separate ways of working reflected the wish of the staff groups to understand their client group, but also to be able to make things better quickly. Surprisingly, and almost perversely, they chose the psychodynamic approach whilst initially believing I could/should help them to "cure" the abusing and, as it quickly emerged, abused parents as well as their abused children within the three to six months of their stay in the unit. They had introjected the referrers' demand that anything other than cure was failure. Within a short time, the conflict generated amongst the staff became very apparent. This conflict emanated from polarized perceptions of all the individual family members as either good or bad, abused or not abused. Adults were stereotyped as parents, whatever "parent" meant to each of the workers. It did not matter whether the parent was a chronological adult or a 16-year-old adolescent with one or more unplanned children. They could not consider the differences between biological facts and object relations. Many of the mainly female staff group also subscribed to the paradigm of men as abusers and could not tolerate the idea, delineated by Estela Welldon (1992), that the women might have participated passively or actively in the abuse. They were clearly unaware that they reacted unconsciously to their male colleagues as abusers, yet they concretely enacted this by being condemnatory when their male colleagues were caught up in transference relationships with abused and abusive residents that were incomprehensible as such to them.

My task seemed formidable. I had to find a way to help them to be able to think about each member of the family unit as a whole person, with a history that was being constantly communicated in their current functioning and modes of relating. I had to convey the concept of the internal as well as the external meaning of behaviour and somehow enable them to think of the parental couple carrying projections for each other and acting them out in projective identification—for example, when abused women repeatedly form relationships with men who abuse their children. Moreover, I needed to help them think in terms of the children's real needs, beyond physical care, and what these children represented in relation to the parents' internal worlds, as well as the impact of abuse on the children's ability to make relationships and their expectations of these.

This was a group of qualified social-work staff, well motivated but without any understanding of unconscious processes (transference, countertransference, projection, projective identification), yet exposed unremittingly to these. They were initially so overwhelmed by each family that they inevitably acted out that which had been projected into them. As the supervisor, I had to be aware of my own countertransference response of feeling like them—that either I had all the answers, or I would be overwhelmed with anxiety about the neediness of each family member and become impotent or act out. On one occasion I found myself also thinking in terms of splitting a family to give each parent and child an ideal parent "somewhere". I became concerned that the staff had become so accustomed to a high level of family dysfunction, including actual abuse, that it ceased to disturb them. They were turning a blind eye (Steiner, 1993, p. 10), thus reflecting and re-enacting the early and current experience of the "parents" as abused children.

This supervision process included, of necessity, some teaching of psychodynamic human growth and development as well as of dynamic processes. It became clear that the most effective medium of supervision was one that focused on the impact on the staff group of the family pathology (or drama). Their enactment of the unconscious processes at work in the families was revealed in the way the workers were, at times, abusive towards each other. This often took the form of a worker being treated by the rest of the staff group as if of no value. The supervisor had to bear the pain of the scapegoated worker being abused by his peers under the guise of professional disagreement. It was as if the worker had no feelings, no humanity. We came to an understanding of this as the scapegoated worker representing the abused child in the family. This was a long, slow process, but they now appreciate how they each carry the different parts of the whole, and they can now utilize this understanding in their work. This team has also modified its aim and now offers a comprehensive assessment period, with a full report to the referrer. This report is valued by referring agencies. By making their task realistically manageable, they have achieved a sense of self-worth and satisfaction, although most staff find the pressure of work at the unit to be such that they leave after about three years. I am now, bar one other, the longest-staying person and as such carry the history of the unit. It is a pleasure to observe how, when new staff members join the unit, the induction process includes the passing-on of their hard-won way of thinking, understanding, and working.

The capacity to endure

I am very aware of how these supervisees have to work with patients who are not usually encountered in private practice, and who are profoundly damaged and damaging. Yet they go on trying, for whatever internal reasons, and bravely seek through supervision an understanding that at one level will help them and, at another level, will make their life more difficult. In the majority of cases, they manage their envy and make good use of whatever is on offer to them. They stay with their patients against all conscious reason, often acting on what they unconsciously recognize.

EXAMPLE

A good example of this arose when a worker presented the case of a young man who unremittingly broke into and damaged cars, resulting in many criminal convictions. She had tried to "discuss" this with him, but, she said, it made no difference. She said that she felt angry and frustrated with him, and yet there was something about him that evoked her concern. He was often at risk of imprisonment, yet she felt compelled to save him from this. Supervision evoked her sense of incomprehension and feelings of being stuck, yet it was also striking how she continued to struggle valiantly to be of assistance. A few minutes before the end of a session she said to me: "It's odd, because he also repairs cars and when he has one to repair he will work night and day without rest or food until it is completed."

I feel this is a rather beautiful example of the worker being unconsciously in touch with the young man's dilemma and with his attempts to resolve his internal conflict through reparation. It was clear that for most of the time she was carrying the reparative aspect for him and that her "speaking up" for him as one who could make good whilst knowing the "destructive him" was important. That is to say, she had unconsciously understood the difference between repetition compulsion—the aim of which is to split and separate objects—and a compulsion to repair.

Supervision contained the worker's and the patient's wish that his damaging and his unsuccessful attempts at reparation might be understood. She appreciated unconsciously that imprisonment, whilst protecting society temporarily, would only reinforce his internal rage and fear of breakdown.

Conclusion

The essence of working with non-analytically trained supervisees is that of bringing to consciousness and making available for thought that which they unconsciously know, and in particular doing this through their countertransference. The risk for them is living with their knowledge, in their setting, with their patients. Then some have to go on to train analytically: their settings are depleted, and the circle of need continues.

CHAPTER SEVEN

(How) Is learning possible in supervision?

Imre Szecsödy

Having been engaged in the training and supervision of psychoanalysts and psychotherapists, and also in the training of supervisors, for many years, I have become increasingly more interested in how learning takes place in supervision. This interest stimulated me to start a study of the supervisory process. My point of departure was that psychoanalysis and dynamically oriented expressive psychotherapy are applications of the same basic science. The aims of both psychoanalysis and psychotherapy are to enable and facilitate change, growth, and emancipation for the troubled individual. The common task is to establish a specific relationship within a specific frame in which the patient can gain insight into his consciously and unconsciously enacted experiences, expectations, wishes, and fears. Appelbaum

---

I wish to express my appreciation to the editors of the following periodicals for giving me permission to use passages from my earlier publications: *Nordisk Psykiatrisk Tidskrift* (1986, 40), *Psychotherapy and Psychosomatics* (1990, 53), *Psychoanalytic Psychotherapy* (1990, 4), *Zeitschrift für psychoanalytische Theory und Praxis* (with H. Kächele & K. Dreyer, 1993, *84*), and *Scandinavian Psychoanalytic Review* (1994, *17*).

(1978) notes that insight presupposes accommodative learning, which goes beyond the assimilative type of learning (defined later in this chapter) and can lead to change, which is further facilitated by what many call a corrective emotional and ideational experience. Within the boundaries of the analytic situation the individual's history is re-experienced, restructured, and, above all, narrated; it acquires new meaning and regains old meanings that were lost. Uniting seemingly separate events into meaningful sequences establishes a coherence, a new order, by way of understanding: "It is a final act of self-appropriation, the appropriation by oneself of one's own history" (Marcus, 1985). (I use the terms psychoanalysis/psychoanalyst and psychoanalytic psychotherapy/psychoanalytic psychotherapist without necessarily distinguishing between the two activities and roles for the purposes of this chapter because my supervision technique and my research investigations were the same in both.)

Art or profession?

In his work, the psychoanalyst and psychotherapist has to take part with his whole personality. He has to follow and understand the conscious and unconscious aspects of the interaction, both cognitively and emotionally, and thus he has to be able to experience and observe at the same time. He has to gain skills in applying specific methods (among them clarifications, confrontations, and interpretations) to facilitate insight. It is no wonder that this work is often compared to that of an artist and is often viewed as a personal attribute rather than one that can be acquired with training (Szecsödy 1990a; Szecsödy, Kächele, & Dreyer, 1993). Training is considered by many to be mainly a process of personal development. In most psychoanalytic institutes senior analysts, who have gained recognition for their theoretical papers, for their lecturing, or for their large analytic practices, become training analysts, which gives them the status and the right to have candidates in training analysis. Working as supervisors follows more or less automatically from this status. Similarly, in psychotherapy training the more experienced therapists take on the responsibility of supervising trainees. Pedagogical competence is neither emphasized nor acknowledged as a prerequisite for working as a supervisor. This may be due to an idealization of analytic work based on the idea that because one has gained an understanding of and skill in the work as such, one has also acquired the capacity to convey this knowledge and skill to others and to facilitate its acquisition by them (Szecsödy, 1994). This idea is also mirrored in the large amount of literature written in an anecdotal manner about supervision, expressing individual and idiosyncratic views as generally valid observations. Even studies that more systematically investigate the supervisory work focus primarily on how one teaches and rather less on how one learns in supervision. It is intriguing that supervision, which is used in all training and at all training institutions, is hardly questioned in regard to its usefulness. There are few studies about the "ill effects" of supervision. Heising (1976) and Sandell (1985) write about the "dysfunction of supervision". Their findings suggest that supervision can have positive effects on therapy outcome generally but not always on the cases that are supervised. I wish to underline that it was not until 1993, at the Sixth IPA Conference of Training Analysts (preceding the 38th Conference of the International Psychoanalytic Association), that the topic of supervision was put into focus. David M. Sachs, the chairman of the organizing committee of that conference, emphasized in his introductory paper that the difficulty of the task of supervision has been greatly underestimated worldwide. Neither training in carrying out supervision nor the study of existing literature was required of new training analysts in most societies!

The place of supervision in a complex "clinical rhombus"

A dictionary definition of supervision is: "An overseeing, surveillance; to inspect, scrutinize, examine; to have control over, to manage, to direct, to conduct." It refers to a situation where psychoanalytic work, carried out by an inexperienced analyst in training, is done under the control and surveillance of a senior (controlling, directing, managing, conducting) analyst. The supervisor as a member of a training institute has not only the status, but also the power and responsibility to judge, evaluate, and influence the status of the candidate/trainee. Another aspect of supervision becomes highlighted by using its Swedish equivalent, *"handledning"*, which means "to lead by the hand", to help a younger, less experienced, less skilled, less knowledgeable colleague, candidate, or trainee to gain knowledge, skill, and experience.

It is important to differentiate supervision according to the trainee's interest in increasing knowledge and skill on the one hand, and acquiring a profession on the other. Depending on which of these two motivations is in the ascendancy, the supervisor may be perceived as a teacher, tutor, mentor, or someone to relate to, rely upon, and identify with; alternatively he might be experienced as judging or controlling in the interest of the trade or the body of professionals, or as a delegate of the "institution". In the latter sense he can be a rival to fight with or one to whom the trainee must submit. Supervisor and trainee can meet in an isolated, secluded room with the intention of working on their task: the trainee to learn, the supervisor to teach. Nevertheless, they are part of the organization in which they work and are influenced by it and are influencing it with more or less realistic expectations and ideas connected with the culturally defined roles and status of the participants. These roles obviously have great potential for satisfying unconscious fantasies and transferential scripts (Szecsödy, 1990a, 1990b, 1990c, 1994; Szecsödy et al., 1993).

Ekstein and Wallerstein (1958) invented the figure and concept of the "clinical rhombus" to describe the mutuality of the intrapsychic and interpersonal influences in the clinical training situation. The trainee's relationship to the supervisor is a composite of intrapsychic expectations and external "realities". "The 'syncretism' of the psychoanalytic education is the problematic combination of roles and functions. The task of the institute is to educate and cure the trainee. The trainee is thus a pedagogic unit or object of teaching and a therapeutic unit or object of psychoanalytic procedure" (Shevrin, 1981). The parties concerned have to deal simultaneously and on different levels with a number of options. Supervisors can be used to defend or defeat a faction, an idea, or a plan or to represent one "school" against another. Institutional rivalry can be channelled through subgroups that form around different supervisors. Conflicts among supervisors in training institutions are frequently expressed through trainees leaving or patients dropping out of treatment. Since they are in a formal organization, the selection of trainees and preconceived notions of what is right and wrong can endanger creativity and paralyse initiative. Clearness of goals and values and the interrelation of tasks are, on the other hand, prerequisites for defining the functions that the individual has to perform and for evaluating the quality of work and competence. The "administrator", in external reality and in the internal representation of rules and ideals, can contribute to development and growth or to fear, submission, secrecy and regression (Szecsödy, 1990a, 1990c).

To show the complexity of these interrelations, I devised the extended clinical rhombus (see Figure 7.1), based on the original idea of Ekstein and Wallerstein. The figure shows how each person or group (patients, families, therapists, supervisors, and their colleagues among trainees and staff) mutually influence the others. All are dependent on, influenced by, and themselves influence the organization they work in. It is pivotal to acknowledge the influence of the organization in which training and work is conducted, as well as to create a platform or setting for working together.

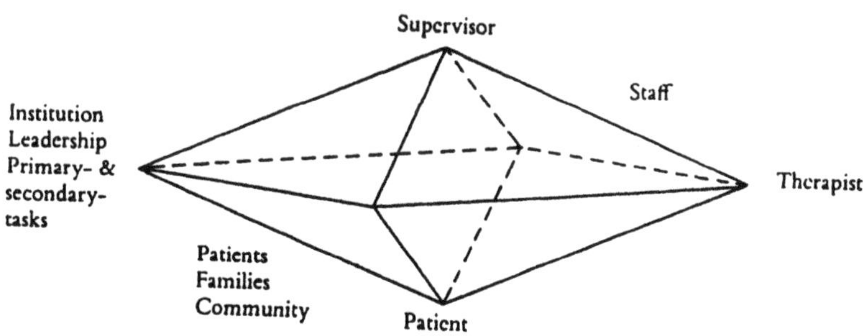

FIGURE 7.1 The extended clinical rhombus (after Ekstein & Wallerstein, 1958). Interactions between patient, therapist, and supervisor are mutually influenced by one another, as well as by other interdependent relationships with staff, other patients, families, administration, the task of the organization, and society outside the institution (Szecsödy, 1986, 1990a).

The task for supervision

According to psychoanalytic theory, the patient is directly and indirectly, manifestly and latently, expressing some wishes, needs, and intentions towards the analyst in the narrative of their interaction. Concomitant with this, the patient expects responses from the analyst as well as from himself, and these often form a repetitive pattern. To recognize and work with these patterns in the analytic interaction is a general aim of psychoanalysis. The unconscious, intentional influence of the analyst in perceiving and selecting these themes has to be acknowledged in the primary interest of the patient.

The task for supervision is to create a setting in which the capacity to learn can develop. To achieve such conditions is not easy and can be complicated by the trainee as well as by the supervisor. How can supervision enhance and safeguard the difficult task of learning, to help the trainee to understand the patient and his own involvement in the intricate interaction that evolves between patient and trainee therapist and between trainee therapist and supervisor? Is there any one way to do it, or are there as many ways as the interactions or even episodes that one studies? This uncertainty is further aggravated by the as yet unanswered question of whether we adjust our working strategies to the particular problems or impose our favourite strategies to confront them. Human understanding and ways of dealing with tasks and problems depend on, are influenced by, and are expressions of mental "structures". Jacob (1981) differentiates between a *cognitive style*, which is a stabilized disposition of perception and cognition; a *working style*, related to the selective use of basic concepts and theories; and the *defensive style*, composed of character traits, transferences, countertransferences, counter-resistances, counter-identifications, and so forth. It is a difficult task to depict these structures and to understand how they aid or hamper the process of learning and teaching (Szecsödy, 1990a, 1994).

There is an ever increasing body of literature about supervision, although I do not wish here to give detailed references. Rather, I present below an integrated picture of what many authors emphasize and agree upon and which corresponds with my own thinking. As in psychoanalysis, it is essential to establish a good "learning alliance" in supervision. This is based on the mutuality of goals in work that are clearly stated as well as experienced by both trainee and supervisor. The supervisor has to be "holding" and "containing" towards the trainee. By holding, I mean the establishment of a phase-specific security in the working relationship; by containing, I mean the provision of an emotional and cognitive "space" to enhance the trainee's recognition and understanding of his conscious and unconscious experiences of interacting with the patient. Langs (1979) emphasized how the keeping of the *frame* in supervision and observing the consequences of breaking it is of crucial importance to be able to comprehend the complex interaction between patient, analyst, and supervisor. Frame has *stationary aspects*, such as agreements on goal, payment, and methods, and general rules for supervision as well as for the supervised therapy; and a *mobile aspect*, which is the continuous reflective review of doing the work together. Among supervisory techniques described in the literature are:

- structuring the supervisory and/or therapeutic interaction directly and indirectly;
- giving information on principles, dynamics, and technique;
- clarifying, by calling the trainee's attention to some gap or ambiguity in his observation and/or understanding;
- reformulating and checking preconceptions;
- confronting the trainee with misconceptions, distortions, warded-off countertransference reactions;
- exploration in relation to content of the ongoing process, or of the ongoing relationship;
- expounding, such as supporting, informing, summarizing; giving general technical or strategic suggestions;
- discussing the formulation of goals for the actual treatment;
- directing the trainee, and prescribing strategies for future sessions.

Only a few publications focus on the vicissitudes of the supervisor/supervisee relationship (Baudry, 1993; Bromberg, 1982; Caligor, 1984; Gross-Doehrman, 1976; Sachs & Shapiro, 1976).

Despite all these descriptions and definitions, too little is understood about the learning process, especially in adults. Fleming and Benedek (1966) reinforced the concept of the "analyst as an instrument", with reference to Freud (1912) regarding the necessity for the analyst to free himself from resistances that would select and distort what he unconsciously perceives. This implies the promise of an unclouded understanding and the risk for idealization. "But whether we like to recognize it or not, I believe all of us have our own (mainly unconscious) hierarchical organization perceiving, screening, measuring the relevance of observational data and finally leading to action for that moment in analysis" (Jacob, 1981). We should add that parallel to the wish to learn and change, there is the fear of the unknown and a tendency to stay with the accustomed and to remain untouched by change.

Learning

Teaching is done and can be studied in *statu nascendi*, and the teacher can be questioned about his aims, intentions, and concerns as well. Learning is more subtle: it is difficult to determine if it has occurred, if it is functional, and if it is an illusory "reduction of cognitive dissonances" (Festinger, 1957).

The following statements can define the main assumptions concerning learning:

- according to a basic psychoanalytic assumption, humans organize their actions to reach certain goals in accordance with their interpretation of a specific situation;
- learning is directed, or at least strongly influenced, by the existing internal structures;
- conscious and unconscious intentions as well as the security principle and the use of psychological defences interfere with the processing of information;
- aspects of learning that are related to imitation and identification are influenced by the quality of object relationships.

The distinctive character of knowledge is organization, dependent on operations belonging to various developmental levels.

In line with Piaget's definition (1958), one expects that trainees learn in two ways: assimilatively and accommodatively. *Assimilative learning* means that the new information is added to the previous, thereby increasing already existing knowledge. The therapist can add newly gained experiences, observations, information, and theory to those he already has, which then become enriched, differentiated, and consolidated. *Accommodative learning* means that encounters with new information result in a fundamental modification of existing cognitive schemata, so that the new encounter can be dealt with. To deal with the information, the trainee must actively engage himself in warding it off or "accommodating" to it by restructuring previously held knowledge, points of view, and theory (Szecsödy, 1990a).

A study of the learning process

In the early 1980s I started a project that had the aims of studying the supervisory process, collecting observations and supplement theories, and clarifying how the trainee learns and the supervisor teaches. I wished to examine the following questions:

- Are there recognizable conditions that could be considered relevant to and optimal for learning?
- Are there recurrent and repetitive patterns that could be differentiated as typical for certain learning problems?
- Does the conduct of supervision differ in any way when dealing with these problems?

These questions all relate to the study of the continuous, sequential interaction between trainee and supervisor. Fifty-six transcripts of recorded supervisory sessions and interviews of supervisors and trainees formed the basis for my descriptive, hypothesis-generating study (Szecsödy, 1990a). After reading transcripts of supervisory sessions, a *"nuclear problem"*—a hypothetical task for the supervisory work—was formulated for each supervisory session on the basis of the following:

1. the quality of interaction between analyst and analysand (as reported by the trainee);
2. the trainee's knowledge and skill in recognizing and understanding the context and/or meaning of this interaction;
3. the way it is presented and worked with in the supervisory session;
4. the quality of interaction between trainee and supervisor.

Inferences were also differentiated according to what type of learning or teaching difficulty was assumed—that is, *lack* or *conflict*. "Lack" meant lack of experience, skill, and knowledge, while "conflict" referred to the defensive avoidance of information. In a similar vein, related to this hypothetical task, an ideal problem-solving route was constructed as a "thought experiment". This described strategies by which the questions and problems might be approached. The route did not describe generalizable rules for supervisory conduct but served only to make explicit what guided the empirical investigator in his observation. Greenburg (1984) suggested the use of Husserl's thought experiment, "by which possible performances are varied freely in imagination, making each observational description a test of the idealized formulation" (p. 142).

I could recognize instances when learning did develop without posing difficulties for the trainee or supervisor, such as when supervisors complemented or completed information the trainees needed and could use, or when trainees rearranged or followed up on observations that helped them to form hypotheses and strategies that seemed relevant and useful within the context of the supervisory session. Notwithstanding, work between trainees and supervisors was often influenced by conflicts connected to the ambiguity and complexity of their task. These findings reconfirmed the necessity to consider the ambiguities in the supervisory relationship:

- The trainee is, more or less, a beginner without much knowledge and/or skill. He has to be open and honest about this in his supervision, as well as with himself. On the other hand, he is expected to be an optimally good therapist for his patient.

- In the therapeutic relationship, the trainee is a "real person", with his professional and personal characteristics, as well as a "transference object" for the patient. As a transference object, he is placed in different and, for him, often foreign, abstruse, or repugnant roles.
- Within the supervisory interaction, the therapist is reconstructing the process he is part of. He is also a trainee who has to expose himself to the supervisor, who aids and teaches but also judges him.
- The supervisor is directly responsible for providing optimal conditions for learning. This has to be correlated with the responsibility that the supervisor has for safeguarding the *patient's* need to receive optimal care (Szecsödy, 1990a; Szecsödy et al., 1993).

One impressive and recurrent finding was that the supervisors less often followed an implicit, consistent, and successive focus than was expected and/or apprehended by them according to their own answers in interviews. Supervisors did not seem to work according to an explicitly or manifestly conceptualized difference between the two kinds of learning problems (lack and conflict as defined above), nor did they adhere to any differentiable strategy to deal with different educational tasks. If they did so intuitively, they seemed to be susceptible to missing the target and changing strategy. Frequently, supervisors seemed to act according to an assumption that giving information was always useful and/or optimal and was, without exception, utilizable by the trainee. They seemed to adhere to this assumption contrary to theories they had about dealing with defences and resistances in the therapeutic interaction. Trainees and supervisors did show some propensity for reacting to the "innate discomfort" of the supervisory situation by becoming abstract or vague, unduly supportive or critical. All trainees retained an insecurity and vulnerability and had a tendency to react defensively. Their learning problem seems always to be connected with their other function, that of interacting therapeutically with their patient (Szecsödy, 1990a, 1990b, 1994; Szecsödy et al., 1993).

It was noticeable that learning did occur most frequently when the supervisor kept an equidistant position. This position is not only an open, non-judgemental, non-competitive attitude, but also includes *the keeping of a continuous and stable focus on the candidate's reconstruction of his interaction with the patient*: in other words, viewing the candidate–patient interaction as a "system" with its own boundaries and frame. In analytic work, we focus on the patient's use of the analyst in his unconscious wishful fantasies and thoughts as they appear in the present—that is, in the transference. The relationship to the analyst is moulded by comprehensive unconscious expectations. As Loewald (1960) emphasized, the patient can discover new material in the object as the analyst fails largely or completely to meet the patient's expectations in certain areas—particularly the area of difficulties—which have previously always been fulfilled by virtue of unconscious steering mechanisms. Similarly, dynamic factors that frequently stimulate conflicts seem always to be present in the supervisory system and influence the learning and teaching process. Nevertheless, it is possible and desirable to maintain the frame and boundaries around both the patient–analyst and the candidate–supervisor systems. For this reason, in addition to the stationary and mobile aspects, I wish to propose a third, a *focusing aspect of frame*. This is the overall and continuous focus that the supervisor has to keep (explicitly or implicitly) on the patient–analyst interaction, assisting the trainee to grasp and connect how this patient's very personality, past experiences, conflicts, and transferential enactments are expressed in the interaction with him, the particular analyst—and how he experiences this, reacts to it, and interacts with the patient, emphasizing aspects of the transference and countertransference (Szecsödy 1990a, 1990c, 1994; Szecsödy et al., 1993).

It is possible, and even advantageous, to define this third aspect of frame-keeping with the help of *boundary maintenance*. Boundaries around the interaction between candidate and supervisor can and have to be maintained by the supervisor through continuous attention on keeping to the primary task. This can serve as a cohesive (not rigid) boundary or frame, enabling the differentiation of intentions, reactions, or interpretations that either belong or are foreign to the two systems. The supervisor has to keep a clear frame by separating his task of doing supervision from that of the candidate, which is to conduct analysis or therapy (Szecsödy, 1990a, 1990c). In recent years, I have also used the phrase "to establish a framework for bloody-serious play", to illustrate the importance of creating a framework for a creative and playful exploration of the trainee's highly complex, profound, and serious work.

In summary, the supervisor has to possess almost innumerable qualities, skills, and knowledge to be able to fulfil the above-mentioned objectives. Outside Sweden, there is hardly any systematic training of supervisors, nor is there any comprehensive textbook available to test or increase the competence of supervisors. This can be taken as expressive of the difficulties in capturing the essential conditions that make learning optimal in supervision, as well as of the irrational, omnipotent, idealizations of the supervisory position.

Training for supervisors

Since 1974, training of supervisors has been undertaken in Sweden by a growing number of organizations and institutions. The curriculum of these training programmes is similar in structure, combining theoretical seminars with the study of the literature and the "super-supervision" of the supervisory work pursued by the trainees for a period of four terms (two years).

The goal of these programmes is to enhance each trainee supervisor's capacity:

- to form a learning alliance with supervisees;
- to focus on the mutually influential interaction between patient and supervisee as well as between supervisee and supervisor;
- to recognize the presence and effect of parallel processes;
- to increase the dexterous use of theory and technique and the capacity for self-reflection and evaluation;
- to encourage the interest for and experience with making tenta-

tive and explicit formulations about the ongoing analytic process, and to recognize transference and countertransference reactions;

- to formulate educational diagnoses, attempting continuously to evaluate the supervisee's difficulties and problems, related both to the lack of knowledge and of skill and to a defensive warding-off of information;
- to recognize the influence and impact of the supervisor's own idiosyncrasies and countertransference reactions on the supervisory process.

The trainees are evaluated according to the following criteria:

1. an ability to establish a platform for "bloody-serious play" that is simultaneously a professional working relationship;
2. an ability to establish a working platform for the supervisor;
3. an ability to use the platform that the super-supervisor was able to establish;
4. an ability to recognize and reflect on the different roles that the supervisor has (a) in the supervisee's institution, (b) in the institution where the supervision is conducted, and (c) in the training institution;
5. an ability to reflect on and understand the supervisor's own motives for undertaking supervision, to differentiate different motives such as the goals of being trained, gaining status, competing, fulfilling illusions, learning about learning;
6. an ability to make a pedagogic diagnosis and, within that diagnosis, differentiate problems due to "lack" from those due to "conflict";
7. an ability to follow and identify the process developing between patient–analyst as well as between trainee–supervisor;
8. an ability to contain and deal with the built-in ambiguities in the supervisory situation, without using primitive defences;
9. a capacity for holding—that is, establishing phase-specific security in the supervisory situation;
10. a capacity for containing—that is, providing space for super-

visees to bring in their emotionally cathected perceptions of the interaction with the patient;

11. an ability to tolerate uncertainties and not-knowing—not forcing the experience to fit preconceived ideas and theories;
12. an ability to explore and to enjoy the "bloody-serious play" of supervision.

Our experiences with the results of the training of supervisors are positive. The Swedish Psychoanalytic Institute arranges training in supervision for those who apply for and are accepted to become training analysts. Only those who received training are permitted to function as supervisors. Similar conditions apply for those who wish to work as a supervisors for trainees of psychoanalytic psychotherapy.

My sincere hope is that by means of conferences on supervision, such as that organized by the EFPP in Toledo and monographs like this one, we can contribute to the growing interest in systematizing knowledge about supervision and in the process of change and learning.

Conclusions

The task of supervision is to create a setting in which the capacity to learn can develop. This is far from easy and can be complicated by factors in both trainee and supervisor. Furthermore, dynamic factors that often provoke conflicts are always present in the supervisory system, and these influence the learning and teaching process. Depending on the trainee's interest in increasing knowledge and skill, the supervisor can be expected to be experienced as a teacher, tutor, mentor, and someone to relate to, rely upon, and identify with. On the other hand, as the trainee is also interested in acquiring professional status, the supervisor might be experienced as judging, controlling in the interest of the trade or the professional association, and a delegate of the "institution." In a study of the learning process, analysing transcripts of supervisory sessions demonstrated that learning occurred most frequently when the supervisor was keeping to a continuous and stable focus on the trainee's reconstruction of his interaction with the patient, viewing the trainee–patient interaction as a "system", with its own boundaries and frame. Boundaries around the interaction between trainee and supervisor can and have to be maintained by the supervisor through continuous attention on keeping to the primary task of helping the trainee to comprehend the nature of the interaction with his patient.

CHAPTER EIGHT

The framework of supervision in psychoanalytic psychotherapy

Robert Langs

All human interactions take place within a framework or context—a setting, an array of rules, and well or poorly defined physical and interpersonal boundaries. Such frames constitute a vital factor in determining the nature and meanings of the interactions that occur within their confines. Thus, transactions involving frames and boundary conditions are, per se, critical events for the individuals involved. These principles, which apply throughout nature, pertain to both psychotherapy and its supervision. (For purposes of focus, I confine my comments here to the supervisory experience; the application of these principles to the treatment situation can be found in Langs, 1992, 1993, 1997.) On both conscious and unconscious levels, ground-rule interventions and behaviours are a major influence on both parties to a supervisory experience. Nevertheless, because of an almost exclusive concentration in supervision on the *contents of presented sessions*, the many powerful effects of *ground-rule–related actions and especially a supervisor's management of the framework of supervision* have been largely neglected.

Clinical work with *the communicative approach to psychotherapy* (Langs, 1992, 1993) and with its supervision (Langs, 1994) has generated a series of observations and precepts that make it imperative to revise our understanding of the key elements of the supervisory process and to redesign its essential techniques. The need for these changes and the means by which they can be explicated are the subjects of this chapter.

Some background considerations

By way of introduction, I briefly summarize the clinical observations and propositions derived from the psychotherapy situation that inform the communicative approach to supervision.

1. *Adaptation* is the most fundamental function of all human organ systems, including the *emotion-processing mind*—the mental module that has evolved to adapt to emotionally charged events or triggers (Langs, 1995, 1996). By adopting a strong adaptive approach to listening to and formulating the material from patients (and their therapists), it has been found that there are two distinct levels of communication within the therapeutic dialogue. The first is direct and manifest, and fraught with evident implications; the second is indirect, latent, and *encoded* in the stories patients tell, usually about events and people outside the therapy.

   a. The adaptation-evoking triggers for a patient's *manifest material* may reside within or outside therapy, but the triggers for *encoded messages* are virtually always constituted by the immediate and recent interventions of the therapist—especially those involving the ground rules and framework of the therapy.

   b. Access to the encoded or deep unconscious meanings of a patient's narratives can be obtained solely through a process called *trigger-decoding*. To carry out this procedure, the stimulus or trigger must be identified and the themes of the displaced or encoded narratives deciphered in light of the meanings of the specific intervention at hand. This effort is very different from working with manifest themes, which are formulated in terms of fantasies and memories. Trigger-decoding stresses unconscious perception and experience, and it involves a deciphering process rather than the extraction of meanings from surface contents.

2. There appear to be two basic systems of the emotion-processing mind: a *conscious system* and a *deep unconscious system*.

a. The conscious system processes contents that are available to awareness either directly or through minimal decoding. This system has evolved to carry out the many adaptations needed for long- and short-term survival, and it tends to be extremely defensive and disinclined to be aware of and deal with most of the potentially disruptive aspects of emotionally charged events, especially threats of harm and death and the *predatory death anxieties they evoke*. In addition, *existential death anxiety*—the universal dread of personal mortality—plays a major role in the defensive alignment of the conscious system, as does the inability of the infant and young child actively to master many aspects of the early traumas they inevitably suffer.

As for rules, frames, and boundaries, the conscious system is frame-insensitive and inclined towards modifications of the ideal ground rules of therapy. There is, indeed, an optimal set of rules of therapy that are universally but *unconsciously sought* by all patients, and they are consistently *validated unconsciously via encoded responses* to therapists' frame-related efforts. The evaluation of the effects of ground-rule interventions, by means of patients' manifest responses and their implications, succumbs to the defensiveness of the conscious system. The result is a failure properly to define the necessary ground of psychotherapy and an inability to appreciate the enormous power and unconsciously mediated consequences of therapists' frame-management efforts.

b. The deep unconscious system relies on unconscious perception for its adaptation-evoking inputs and engages in deep unconscious processing to arrive at adaptive responses that are, in the emotional realm, far more constructive than those reached by the conscious mind. Nevertheless, the conscious system is unable to utilize this deep wisdom because it reaches awareness only in encoded form—the meanings to which it responds are profoundly anxiety-provoking.

Through its encoded themes, the deep unconscious system reveals an unswerving wish for, and support of, frame-securing interventions. Encoded themes, properly trigger-decoded in light of a therapist's frame-related interventions, also recognize and respond to the harmful effects of frame modifications (Langs, in press). On the whole, frame management is far more effective when based on trigger-decoding than it is when patients' manifest and implied responses are used for guidance.

Implications for supervision

The communicative approach to, and understanding of, psychotherapy supervision is radically different from approaches based on classical models of psychoanalytic and psychodynamic thinking. The essential differences lie with the following:

1. The recognition of two levels of supervisory efforts and experience: *conscious system supervision* and *deep unconscious system supervision*.

   a. Conscious system supervision involves the cognitive teaching efforts of the supervisor and is focused on the material from the presented psychotherapy sessions and the supervisee's manifest responses to the supervisor's teaching efforts. In this regard, communicative supervision stresses the use of trigger-decoding and *encoded unconscious validation* of all interventions—those of the supervisee with the supervised patient, and those of the supervisor in the teaching situation (material is presented sequentially and teaching is done in a predictive manner: Langs, 1994). Thus, frame-related interventions are treated as especially important aspects of the therapeutic experience of both the supervised patient and the supervisee.

   b. Deep unconscious system supervision involves exposing the unconscious experiences of both parties to supervision and is centred around the supervisor's management of the ground rules of the supervisory situation and the supervisee's frame-related behaviours as they pertain to the supervision. This level of supervisory intervention is critical to the learning experience of the supervisee because the deep unconscious system is focused on perceiving and adapting to the events occurring in its immediate interactions and setting; in supervision, this is the supervision rather than the supervised therapy situation.

This realm of experience takes place outside awareness (unless it is trigger-decoded), has strong effects on the supervisee's (and supervisor's) interventions with patients (and personal lives), and is disruptive to the teaching efforts of the supervisor if it contradicts his conscious teaching efforts. In all, then, while both levels of supervisory work need to be soundly and validly conducted, a supervisee's actual here-and-now, deep unconscious experiences with a supervisor are far more crucial to the effects of supervision than the surface teaching that occurs through a discussion of the case material from sessions that take place outside the supervisory setting. Indeed, secured frames are the *sine qua non* for valid and deeply effective supervisory teaching efforts.

2. There are three common means through which supervisees and/or supervisors may communicate their deep unconscious experiences of a supervisory interaction.

a. The first is through a supervisee's selection of a case for presentation. Patients are chosen for a variety of conscious reasons—for example, they are difficult to treat or there is a crisis in the therapy. But there are, as well, critical unconscious reasons for this choice. On the one hand, the presented material contains narrative themes that encode the supervised patient's unconscious perceptions of the supervisee's therapeutic efforts. In this regard, deep unconscious guilt is a common motivating force in supervisees' selection of material in that the need is to reveal the errors of their ways. In addition, supervisees unwittingly select cases for presentation in order to recruit their patients' narrative themes as vehicles for conveying their own unconscious experiences of the supervision, especially their unconscious perceptions of the supervisory settings and ground rules as defined by their supervisors (Korn & Carmignani, 1987). This level of interaction and impact takes place without awareness interceding, unless trigger-decoding is applied to the material at hand.

b. The second common means of conveying deep unconscious messages within the supervisory situation involves the *coincidental stories* told by either party to the supervision. This vehicle for encoded communication includes all narrative departures from the material under study, such as references to other patients, supervisors, or supervisees, and all types of personal and other stories. These tales may be told for a variety of conscious reasons and may be well rationalized as relevant to the teaching situation. However, they are exquisitely selected by the deep unconscious system to convey critical and immediately relevant unconscious perceptions of current triggering events and their unconsciously experienced meanings. Not surprisingly, the themes in these displaced and encoded tales almost always pertain to ground-rule issues and impingements—the realm to which the conscious system is least sensitive.

c. The third means of conveying unconscious messages involves the rules, frames, and boundaries of the supervisory situation. The management of the framework of supervision is primarily the responsibility of the supervisor. However, supervisees also have impact on the frame. For example, they may request a reduction in the fee for supervision—a frame modification—or may ask a supervisor who has requested a change in the time of the supervision to keep the present time, which is a frame-securing intervention by a supervisee in response to a supervisor's efforts to modify the frame. The deep unconscious meanings of these frame-related activities will be found in the narratives that accompany such efforts.

The deep unconscious level of education has a most compelling effect on the supervisee, and it strongly, though unconsciously, affects his or her approach to doing psychotherapy. While *cognitive education* is being offered manifestly and consciously, *emotional education* is being offered latently and deeply unconsciously—and no matter how incisive the direct teaching, a more powerful form of teaching is going on indirectly. There is no possible other way that a supervisor can influence the critical deep unconscious experience of a supervisee except through his management of the framework of the supervision and through trigger-decoding the encoded narratives that the supervisee (or supervisor) communicates in the course of the supervisory work.

In general, supervisors should refrain from introducing their own stories into a supervision. The tale itself is a self-revelation, and the frame break is compounded when the story involves another patient—a violation of the total confidentiality of that patient's therapy. In addition, these narratives are filled with encoded meanings that are unconsciously perceived by the supervisee, even though neither party is aware of their presence. Teaching that occurs entirely without awareness by either party is almost always destructive to all concerned—the encoded messages are usually quite disruptive.

One other point: until now, psychoanalysts have stressed individual differences at the expense of the underlying, species-specific universals on which these differences are grounded. Conscious system supervision tends to focus on the distinctive features of a given patient–therapy dyad, and the seeming need for flexibility when it comes to the ground rules. In contrast, deep unconscious system supervision addresses basic universals and then explores how each individual patient (and supervisee and supervisor) employs them. It also recognizes the universal need for secured frames as reflected in encoded narratives, despite the great variability of conscious system attitudes in this regard. Universals individually adhered to is the essential finding (Langs, 1996).

The ideal ground rules of supervision

Consciously, the ideal framework for supervision is all but impossible to define—manifest individual preferences vary enormously. On the other hand, it is quite feasible to define the ideal, *unconsciously validated*, universally sought framework for the supervision of psychotherapy because deep unconscious frame needs are consistent across individuals and inherent to the architecture of the emotion-processing mind. The ideal ground rules for supervision are not unlike the ideal framework of psychotherapy (Langs, 1992, in press). Essentially, the optimal supervisory frame includes:

1. A totally private and professional setting with an effectively sound-proofed office.
2. A private referral of the supervisee to the supervisor, and the absence of prior personal or professional contact between them.
3. A single setting for the supervision, with a set fee, a defined length and frequency of sessions, and a fixed appointment time (usually once weekly for forty-five or fifty minutes).
4. Complete privacy and confidentiality for the supervision, with no recording of any aspect of the supervisory presentation or teaching experience by either party to the supervision. Thus, for both the supervised therapy and the supervision itself, there are no process notes, tape-recorded or videotaped sessions, or jottings of any kind made by either party to the supervision. Similarly, no reports on the supervisory work are made to others, nor are evaluations or assessments released to third parties.
5. A reconstruction by the supervisee of the therapy hour under supervision from memory and in strict sequence without the use of notes.
6. The instruction and other comments offered by the supervisor to be based entirely on the material of the session under consideration in a given supervisory hour. Both parties to the supervision refrain from extraneous comments, including anecdotes and stories of a personal or professional nature. In particular, neither supervisor nor supervisee should allude to colleagues, friends, relatives, or other patients—the supervision is concerned exclusively with the material from the sessions with the patient whose therapy is under supervision.
7. The relative anonymity of both the supervisor and supervisee. This means that there are no personal revelations and no offer of personal opinions or suggestions, other than those needed

for purposes of teaching and learning in connection with the reported case material. All comments on both sides closely adhere to the presented material and its implications—and the interventions they call for. In all, then, the teaching and learning is based entirely on the material from the sessions with the supervised case.

8. Confinement of the contacts and interactions between supervisor and supervisee to the supervisory setting and to the allotted time. The relationship is maintained entirely on a professional level, without gratuitous favours or shifts to other types of interacting and relating.
9. There is no physical contact between the parties to the supervision except for a handshake at the beginning and end of the supervision.
10. All teaching efforts to be carried out in predictive fashion and subjected to a search for encoded validation. All of the interventions that have a bearing on supervision—whether from the supervisor or the supervisee (to his patient or, on occasion, to the supervisor)—should be confirmed unconsciously by means of encoded narratives. The relevant imagery may come from the presented case material or from a coincidental narrative told by the supervisee—or unthinkingly by the supervisor. Most importantly, every significant teaching assessment and recommendation made by a supervisor must find encoded confirmation in the subsequent material from the supervised patient before it can be considered to be correct. Supervision is not conducted by fiat; the encoded communications from the supervised case is the final arbiter of the validity of a supervisor's teachings.

There are, of course, very few supervisory experiences that have been or are presently being conducted within the ideal framework for supervision as universally validated by deep unconscious systems. Nevertheless, compromised settings and ground rules and modifications to the frame during a supervisory experience not only interfere with conscious learning, they also unconsciously direct and motivate supervisees to use interventions that are harmful to their patients—and to themselves as well.

Modified and compromised frames for supervision unconsciously pressure supervisees to make erroneous verbal interventions, to miss important interpretive opportunities, and to sustain inappropriate silences (i.e. to miss indicated interventions). Most tellingly, a supervisor's frame deviations also teach and motivate supervisees to do such things as mismanage the ground rules and frameworks of the therapies they conduct, select personal therapists who are frame-deviant and unconsciously harmful, and destructively modify frames in their daily lives.

Supervisors' frame modifications virtually always evoke frame modifications by their supervisees—frame deviations beget frame deviations and become a basic but maladaptive way of coping and living. Often, a vicious circle is established in which a supervisor's frame breaks lead to frame modifications by the supervisee, which prompts further frame modifications by the supervisor, and so on. When a frame-deviating personal therapist is added to the supervisee's life, there is a strong likelihood of a career as a frame-deviant psychotherapist.

The heritage created in this way is damaging to all concerned. The supervisee engages in maladaptive frame modifications in his professional and private lives, and the supervisor experiences *deep unconscious guilt* for the harm his frame deviations are causing the supervisee. This in turn leads the supervisor to engage in further maladaptive and self-punitive frame breaks that are unconsciously designed for self-punishment and the temporary amelioration of the related unconscious guilt. A great deal of suffering by supervised patients, supervised therapists, and supervisors themselves arises from the frame modifications that occur in supervision; their unconsciously mediated effects are quite strong and very real.

Documenting the effects of the supervisory frame

A major part of the problem in appreciating the deep unconscious effects of the frame-management efforts of a supervisor arises from the essential nature of the supervisory experience. In psychotherapy, the main source of validation of therapists' interventions lies with patients' encoded narratives, as they speak for the presence or absence of deep unconscious confirmation. This type of indirect and entirely unconscious validation is the only presently known reliable means through which a therapist can evaluate the effects of his interventions. The conscious system is so highly defensive and self-punitive in its assessments (Langs, 1995, 1996) that direct responses to an intervention are an exceedingly unreliable basis for these evaluations. Only the deep unconscious system has the wisdom and non-defensive adaptive insight to appraise properly the accuracy and helpfulness of a therapist's efforts—be they silences, verbalized interpretations and other comments, or frame-management efforts.

In therapy, this assessment tool depends on the narratives from patients that emerge in the course of free associating. Patients are almost certain, by nature, to respond to frame alterations (securing or deviating) with encoding stories that reflect their unconscious assessment and adaptation to these triggering events. As a result, a psychotherapist usually has the material needed to interpret and understand the deep unconscious meanings of his currently active frame-related interventions. All that is required is the therapist's ability to trigger-decode the patient's narrative themes—to decipher their disguised meanings in light of the most recent frame-deviant or frame-securing interventions.

The situation is quite different in supervision because the supervisee is not required to—and should not—free associate. While the selection of a case for supervision typically encodes important unconscious perceptions of the supervisor and the frame that he is offering to the supervisee, there are few appropriate opportunities for supervisees to narrate in response to a supervisor's frame-related interventions. On occasion, a supervisee nevertheless will offer a spontaneous, marginally related story, a narrative that departs from the material of the case presentation. This story most certainly will encode significant unconscious perceptions of the supervisor's teaching efforts and frame-management interventions, and they can be trigger-decoded for both insight and, where needed, rectification of the deviant frame.

Similarly, a supervisor may think of a narrative of some kind, be it about another patient, a personal life event, or anything else in storied form. This narrative should be privately decoded in light of the prevailing frame-related triggers to enable the supervisor to grasp the deep unconscious issues raised by his frame-management efforts, or by a frame-related action by the supervisee.

These principles apply to both frame-modifying and frame-securing interventions. The latter is illustrated, for example, by a shift made from a clinic to a private setting or when a policy of randomizing the time of the supervisory meetings is changed so that a single set time is established. Encoded validation consistently follows this type of frame change—along with the emergence of notable secured-frame anxieties as well (see below).

A new mode of supervision

There is, as expected, a standard model of communicative supervision that adheres to the ground rules and principles described above. However, a second form of communicative supervision was developed in response to the difficulties in gaining access to the critical deep unconscious experiences of supervisees in the immediate supervisory situation. It is called *self-processing supervision* (Langs, 1994), and it combines communicative psychotherapy (Langs, 1993) with the supervisory work.

The therapy aspect of this modality is designed to afford the greatest possible access to a supervisee's deep unconscious experience by obligating him to begin each session with a dream or made-up story and to generate extended narrative *guided associations* to the dream elements. This is followed with the identification of both the supervisee's and the supervisor's impingements on the framework of the supervision—respectively termed *self-indicators* and *the adaptation-evoking triggering events*. The exploration is completed when the triggers are linked to the narrative themes, which are then trigger-decoded to reveal the supervisee's deep unconscious perceptions and processing of these frame-related events.

The supervisory part of this process follows. It, too, is carried out according to communicative principles and includes the requisite of validation of all supervisory interventions through responsive encoded narratives from supervisees and their patients.

Given that the frame-related deep unconscious experiences of the supervisee have significant unconscious effects on his therapeutic work and personal life, the development of a paradigm within which these experiences and their specific effects on a supervisee's work with patients can be identified and worked through is of considerable value. Since the deep unconscious system of the emotion-processing mind is activated entirely by events in the immediate situation, there is no other presently known effective means of accessing and bringing into awareness this level of experience. Efforts to do so in a supervisee's personal psychotherapy cannot work, because the encoded narratives that the supervisee reports to his therapist pertain to the *therapist's* frame-management efforts and not to the supervisory situation. It is possible consciously to discuss frame issues about another situation, but it is not possible to access the deep unconscious experience of these issues except through immediately activated encoded narratives and their themes.

The role of death anxiety

There are, of course, many unconscious motives for the neglect by psychotherapists of *encoded* communications and the ground rules of psychotherapy and its supervision. Secured supervisory frames, in which the ideal ground rules are established and maintained, are ego- and self-enhancing and fully support a supervisor's valid teaching efforts. They provide a supervisee unconsciously with a model of a supervisor of great capability, strength, and wisdom, who is thereby inherently available for constructive unconscious introjective identifications.

Securing the ground rules of supervision also speaks for active and effective forms of secured-frame adaptation, without pathological defensiveness and inappropriate satisfactions. This approach entails a supervisor's renunciation of his own pathological needs and defences in the service of the educational needs of the supervisee and the therapeutic needs of the supervised patient. All in all, a supervisor who can create a secured frame for supervision offers an optimal set of conditions for the enduring and sound education of the supervisee.

Why, then, have supervisors failed to appreciate and advocate secured frames?

One of the most compelling reasons for this oversight lies with the realization that, in addition to their enhancing qualities, secured frames create enormously dreaded, deep unconscious *existential death anxieties* that pertain to the inevitability of personal demise (Langs, 1997). These universal anxieties are among the most dreaded of human experiences, and in supervision they stem from the sense of relative immobility, constraint, and entrapment that is inherent to secured-frame situations. This form of death anxiety, which usually operates outside awareness, is difficult to tolerate and adapt to largely because it can never be fully mastered.

Situations that arouse existential death anxieties are especially unbearable in individuals with significant histories of early- and later-life death-related traumas, and in those dealing with current death-related events. The frequency with which humans experience such traumas, and the general human pessimism regarding our ability to deal with the inevitability of personal death, account for the extent to which supervisors and their supervisees tend to prefer modified frames to secured frames. Given that no one can successfully overcome this eventuality, defences that deny death—and frame modifications are chief among these defences—are much preferred to adapting to these issues in as best a secured-frame fashion as possible.

Within limits, denial of death is an adaptive psychological mechanism that enables humans to cope with the challenges of life without being overwhelmed by death anxiety and preoccupations with personal mortality. Healthy denial finds behavioural support in situations like celebrations, festivals, sporting events, and other manic-like activities that cause no harm and bring relief to those involved. Nevertheless, all forms of denial restrict and interfere with learning and effective adaptation; the invocation of denial mechanisms always entails a measure of penalty.

The single most common yet unappreciated form of behavioural denial involves departures from the ideal ground rules of a given situation and relationship—escapes from secured frames. The rule breaker unconsciously believes that he is an exception to all rules, especially the fundamental existential rule of life—that death is its inevitable outcome. Whatever their conscious justification, necessary and unnecessary supervisory frame deviations serve to deny existential death anxieties, especially those that are activated by secured frames.

Frame modifications offer broad, but costly, pathological forms of gratification and defense and, specifically, operate as maladaptive ways of denying death. They involve obliterations of reality and intrapsychic experience and therefore inevitably interfere with the education of the supervisee. Modifying frames is a basic, maladaptive mode of adaptation that precludes healthy coping, for which secured frames are a vital necessity. Thus, a supervisor's use of this type of denial-based defense against existential death anxieties unconsciously becomes a maladaptive model for the coping efforts of a supervisee—within and outside of his therapeutic work. Modifying frames becomes a way of life and a heritage passed on from supervisor to supervisee and eventually to his supervisees and patients as well.

There is, however, another quality of supervisory frame deviations that unconsciously wreaks havoc with supervisees: *frame modifications are always persecutory—they evoke unconscious experiences of assault and harm, and of predatory forms of death anxiety* (Langs, 1997). In modifying a supervisory frame, the supervisor moves the supervisee out of the frying-pan (having to deal with secured-frame, existential death anxieties) into the fire (having to deal with deviant-frame, predatory death anxieties). These latter unconscious anxieties generally prompt supervisees to utilize persecutory interventions with their patients. Typically, these unconsciously activated interventions then evoke criticism by the supervisor, who is unaware that he has unconsciously created the motivation for these harmful efforts—another aspect of the vicious circles created by frame modifications.

Some final perspectives

There are many implications to the findings and ideas alluded to in this chapter. In terms of fundamental efforts at adaptation, it is clear that patients, supervisees, and supervisors consciously, though not deeply unconsciously, prefer denial-based frame modifications, however persecutory, in lieu of secured frames and their activation of existential death anxieties, however enhancing they may be. The deep lack of faith in humans regarding their ability to cope effectively with personal mortality has proven to be fateful for both psychotherapy and its supervision. The cost involved in harm to all concerned is enormous, but it goes unrecognized and largely denied.

In practical terms, private-practice supervisors are in a position to create the ideal conditions for supervision, and they should do so. This action, however, requires an understanding and mastery of a supervisor's own existential death anxieties and a willingness to forego working with potential supervisees with whom a secured supervisory frame is impossible—for example, those who have been patients of the supervisor, those with whom the supervisor has had prior contact, and referrals from other supervisees or from patients of the supervisor.

Perhaps the most difficult type of situation to resolve effectively is one in which the supervision is conducted under the auspices of a training institute or programme. The best solution available at the moment appears to be allowing supervisees to select a supervisor from a roster of certified supervisors, and for the supervision to be conducted on a private basis without reports on the supervisee to any outside party. The supervisee's graduation from or certification by the training programme would then depend on case presentations to a committee of the institute from which the supervisee's therapist and supervisor are excluded. This approach respects the critical finding that frame-related actions have far greater effects on supervisees than supervisors' verbal teachings.

Finally, it is well to appreciate that supervision based on the communicative approach is dramatically different from that based on any other theoretical foundation. The realization that the deep unconscious system of the emotion-processing mind responds to each and every intervention made by a supervisor, the recognition of the primacy of unconscious adaptation, and the use of trigger-decoding enable supervisors and supervisees to enter and process a world of deep unconscious experience that is otherwise obscured. Trigger-decoding shows psychotherapy supervision in a highly distinctive light and calls for many revisions in how supervision is currently practiced. Perhaps most critical among these changes is the need to understand and properly secure the ground rules and framework of the supervisory situation to the greatest extent feasible.

Frame must be dealt with before content; meaningful content is evoked by frame-related transactions—and both maxims deserve our full respect.

CHAPTER NINE

An advanced training in the supervision and teaching of psychotherapy

Kurt Gordan

The training of psychotherapists can never be better than the competence of its supervisors. In 1976, this realization influenced those of us working at the Erica Foundation to plan and put into action the first two-year systematic supervisor training programme for psychotherapists in Sweden. [The Erica Foundation in Stockholm, Sweden, is an independent institute providing at university level: (1) a professional training for child and adolescent psychotherapists; (2) a psychotherapy service for children and adolescents; and (3) research. Both the training programmes and the psychotherapy service are based on psychodynamic approaches. The institute is largely funded by central government and the county council.]

During the twenty years that have passed since then, this training has naturally changed and improved. However, the overall

This chapter is an expanded version of Chapter 7 in Kurt Gordan, *Psychotherapy Supervision in Education, Clinical Practice and Institutions.* Northvale, NJ: Jason Aronson, 1996.

plans and content have, for the most part, proved to be practicable in reaching the goals that we set out to achieve. Our model for the training of supervisors and teachers of psychotherapy has also formed the basis for the majority of training courses for supervisors that have now been arranged elsewhere in Scandinavia. Considering the great interest that our training for supervisors has aroused outside Scandinavia, it is appropriate to describe here the essence of the Erica Foundation training for supervisors and teachers of psychotherapy.

The training goal

From its conception the supervision training programme has had three goals:

1. Overall, to provide an advanced training that gives the participants the competence to conduct supervision for those training to become specialist-level psychodynamic psychotherapists. This means a psychotherapy training that leads to full state certification in Sweden for psychotherapists and in which being supervised is included as a compulsory unit.

This goal is founded on the conviction that competence as a psychotherapist is a necessary but insufficient prerequisite for shouldering the role of a supervisor who is "good enough". Our experience has taught us that some outstanding therapists may function badly as supervisors. Thus the goal was to develop skills in the supervisor trainees that lead to a professional identity as a supervisor alongside the psychotherapist identity they brought with them.

2. To design the training programme in such a way that it also gives the participants competence to supervise students in lower-level psychotherapy trainings and to supervise psychotherapists and other staff in health care and treatment institutions.

The need for qualified supervisors for the Erica Foundation's own psychotherapy training, and for equivalent programmes in Sweden, was the incentive for building up this programme. There was and is, however, also an urgent need for supervisors for the staff of health-care establishments and for treatment personnel at institutions for children and adolescents, and so on.

3. To impart knowledge concerning the teacher's role and didactics in respect of psychotherapy training. Its objective is that the participants themselves will be able to function as teachers of psychotherapy, psychoanalytic theory, and so forth, subjects in which emotional receptivity is a prerequisite for real and effective learning.

There is a shortage of highly qualified psychotherapists in Sweden. The majority of those who participate in supervisory training have experienced pressure at their work places to take on duties as teachers within the framework of various psychotherapy training programmes. It is, moreover, reasonable to expect that psychotherapy supervisors, who have had the benefit of long-term, advanced training, should share their know-how.

After decades of experience with the training of psychoanalysts and psychotherapists, it is relatively clear at the present time what theoretical elements should be part of the courses. However, we still have very inadequate information as to how such content should best be structured so that it leads to "emotional learning". Naturally, this problem has blocked the development of the teaching portion of the training. Even though there has been some development of pedagogical elements, their part in the teacher-and-supervisor training is altogether still too limited.

The training design

Admission requirements

Training for supervisors has been open to full state-certified psychotherapists with at least two years of psychotherapy practice post-certification. Personal suitability for supervision and teaching is assessed through interviews. The majority of applicants have been very well qualified psychotherapists. They have had considerably experience as psychotherapists and have often worked as supervisors for varying periods of time. A well-integrated identity as a psychotherapist has proved to be an important prerequisite if the student is to be able to profit from this training.

Training has been open to applicants from the whole country. In keeping with the aims of the Erica Foundation, applicants with experience in child and adolescent psychotherapy have been given preference. The fact that participants have a mixture of backgrounds—basic education in psychiatry, psychology, or psychiatric social work, and either child or adult psychotherapeutic training and experience in various fields of activity—has proved to be a great asset in discussions in the supervision groups as well as in seminars. When it is a matter of extremely well-qualified course participants, as in this training, heterogeneity in the groups is probably a benefit rather than a disadvantage.

Structure

The course is monitored and organized by a training committee. Every intake includes twelve participants. Training originally lasted only three terms, but after a few years this was increased to four. The main reason for this extension was that it often proved to be difficult or impossible in three terms for the therapists to conclude their therapies and for the supervisors to work through and conclude their supervisions. There is no doubt that in a training situation it is important for therapists and supervisors to have the opportunity to work within the framework of their supervisions, starting with the selection of patients suitable for insight therapy, followed by evolution of the therapy itself, and finally attending to separation issues. In addition, the extension to two years opened up chances for increased pedagogical training of the participants as seminar leaders.

The scheduled tuition is concentrated on half a day per week. In addition to this, the programme includes independent study and supervision tasks.

The training includes the following three elements:

1. theoretical instruction;
2. supervising cases;
3. supervising the supervision.

Theoretical instruction

Theoretical instruction is given in seminar form with a frequency of two sessions a week. During the greater part of the first year, it is mainly the teachers and the guest lecturers who are responsible for the instruction. Later on, during the second year, the course participants themselves are each responsible for two seminars.

Considering the participants' own skill and clinical experience, and for pedagogical reasons, we have made it our practice to limit the number of external lecturers and place the responsibility for the content and form of seminars to a great extent on the participants themselves. Nevertheless, it has been the course leader's overriding responsibility to make sure that the pivotal questions of the training are dealt with in one form or another during the progress of the course.

During the entire training period, participants rotate the tasks of writing *short summaries* of lectures and seminars. These are copied and distributed to the participants as well as to course administration personnel and the leaders of the supervision groups. They serve an important function in communication between all parties concerned and in the coordination of the teaching.

Participants' own seminars. These occupy a central position in the student teachers' training. Every participant chooses, in consultation with the course leader, a subject related to the theory and application of supervision or to pedagogical questions and is thereafter completely responsible for the planning and implementation of two seminars.

The course leader is available to the participants for advice on planning and for suggestions about suitable literature. It is also the course leader's task to coordinate the seminars, as far as possible, with regard to content and focus so that, for example, seminars dealing with ethical matters, parallel processes, or supervision at health care institutions follow each other in a logical order. In addition, the course leader is often obliged to assist the participants in focusing on issues that deal with supervision or pedagogy and to help them refrain from the temptation to devote time to psychotherapy matters already familiar to them.

A member of the training committee is present at the first seminar, and his primary task is to observe the lecturer's presentation and the reactions of the participants. The final twenty minutes of the seminar's double period are reserved for a survey of that seminar leader's performance from the pedagogical angle. The course participant/seminar leader changes hats with the member of the training committee, who now takes command of the seminar. The ideas of the participants and the training committee member about the seminar leader's performance, the quality of contact with his listeners, his use of material and time, his receptivity to ideas—in short, the whole pedagogical process—are reviewed and discussed. In this context, and as an introduction to the discussion, it is important to take into account the seminar leader's own perception of his teacher role. Did he think he had succeeded in conveying his message? Had he achieved his goal for the seminar? Was he disturbed or stimulated by his participants' remarks? Comparing the seminar leader's subjective perceptions with the impressions of the participants often proves instructive.

The participant's second seminar is usually devoted to delving deeper into the subject he had chosen for the first. By now, the practical experience that he gained as a trainee supervisor has increased.

Participants have been in agreement about the value of the participation of the training committee member as a pedagogical observer and discussion leader during the first seminar. On the other hand, during the second seminar there are sometimes divergent opinions about the value of our model. The organization of the training programme, after all, has been marked by efforts to let the participants successively take over the responsibility for the teaching. It might seem logical for the seminar participants to be completely responsible for both the content and the pedagogical analyses of the seminars. On the other hand, there is an obvious risk that the pedagogical focus and learning would be lost in the absence of a teacher from outside the student group. The group would be vulnerable to being captivated by the *content* of the seminar and might be tempted to avoid critical views of their associate's performance as a teacher.

One problem with our model for pedagogical training has been that the participants often thought that the time for this training infringed on the time for discussion of subject *content*, so that the latter was far too circumscribed. In the face of this criticism it may be argued that the goal for the seminars, alongside the pedagogical objective, is to provoke hypotheses and debate about styles of teaching and to stimulate the participants' ideas, rather than to bring discussion of the subject matter to a conclusion or solution.

Over the years it has become apparent that many extremely skilful and experienced psychotherapists completely lack experience as lecturers and avoid the teacher role as much as possible. For these persons especially, conducting their own seminars during the training has been a profound and beneficial experience, and in several cases they have now begun to accept teaching assignments. For other participants, too, it has been important for them to get a picture of their own presentations and to have feedback from a competent group under relatively secure conditions. It has also been our experience again and again that the pedagogical skills of the participants showed a remarkable improvement from the first of their own seminars to their second.

Content of the theoretical instruction and study of the literature. This is based on the compulsory textbook, *Psychotherapy Supervision in Education* (Gordan, 1996). In addition, lecturers and seminar leaders refer to other relevant articles and books (e.g. Bernard & Goodyear, 1992; Mackinnon, 1986; Mackinnon, Glick, & Neutzel, 1986; Minnes, 1987; Styczynski, 1980).

During the first term, it is normal for the teachers to provide basic information about the history of supervision, definitions of concepts and goals, and the demarcation between supervision and therapy, supervision and consultation, and so forth. The participants are expected to enter more deeply into these subjects in the seminars that they lead themselves. During the first period, when the participants also begin to be supervised in their own supervision, it is important to take up questions concerning the conditions for therapy and supervision, introductory interviews, the design of frames and contracts, legal and ethical aspects of the supervisor's responsibility, and so on.

During the second and third terms, the instruction leads to a deeper knowledge of theoretical concepts and the methodology of supervision. The participants are now prepared for their task as seminar leaders by attending a teacher-led series on "Pedagogy in Psychotherapist Training", and discussions take place about the pedagogical organization of the seminars. Once the participants have chosen the subjects for their seminars, it is possible for the training committee to see to the design of the total content of the course and arrange supplementary lectures—for example, in subjects like the supervision of psychotherapies with psychotic patients, the significance of the supervisor's gender, conflicts between student and supervisor, group processes in supervision groups, and so forth.

To provide a more vivid impression of the content of the seminars, the following are two brief examples of important issues that regularly give rise to intensive discussion in seminar groups.

1. Considering that it is generally accepted that the first meeting is of great importance in developing a therapeutic relationship, it is remarkable that the question of how the supervisor introduces himself to the supervisee has scarcely been discussed in the literature.

When we want to build a friendship or relationship in our private lives, we start with the assumption that mutuality and an exchange of thoughts and feelings form the basis for such a relationship. When a psychoanalyst or a psychotherapist initiates a collaboration with a new patient, he is essentially expressing the opposite approach. He strives to be as anonymous as possible regarding his own person and his private life. His primary goal with this "neutral" attitude is to facilitate the patient's projections of earlier experiences and the development of a transference neurosis. But to what extent does a *supervisor* wish to stimulate transference and regression in his student? A comrade type of relationship, on the other hand, where transference is definitely opposed, may be tempting to a young and insecure supervisor. However, it can hardly be the basis for process-focused supervision, and in difficult and anxiety-filled situations it is of little use to the student. It may be difficult for the supervisor to find the optimal distance for the learning process.

2. Many authors emphasize the importance of paying attention to the student's emotional reactions in the treatment situation and of helping him to become aware of his blind spots. At the same time they warn against seeking to meet the student's need for psychotherapy within the framework of supervision. This view can be supported theoretically and may serve as an excellent goal in the work of the supervisor. In practice, however, the majority of supervisors find themselves in situations where supervision has imperceptibly passed over into psychotherapy—a development that was probably not the goal of either of the parties.

The following case history illustrates a situation so common that the majority of supervisors will probably recognize themselves in it.

> Eva, in her 40s, was in supervision with me. Her therapy patient was also a woman in her 40s. Both had rather similar life styles: academic education, a small house in the suburbs, children in the latency period, and husbands established in their careers. After about a year of therapy, the patient went to a week-long conference. She was intellectually very stimulated, fell in love with a fellow course participant, and came home to sail right into a painful marital crisis. She saw her husband with new eyes, and aggressively questioned her whole way of running her life. She now wanted "self-fulfilment" and to utilize her own resources. The patient's anxiety-driven actions aroused extremely strong emotions in Eva, who was experiencing a similar life-crisis. Now, too, Eva's own marriage was called into question. Earlier problems came to the fore: dependency, aggressiveness and guilt toward an overprotective mother, and certainly questions about her female identity.

> Eva had been in psychoanalysis many years earlier. It was obvious to both the supervisor and the supervisee that she was now in need of renewed therapy or analysis. But it was soon apparent that she would have to wait at least a year before a vacancy; in addition, she did not have any notion of how she was going to pay for therapy. But the need was acute: the complex of problems affected not only Eva's private life, but also the psychotherapy and supervision. Eva became inhibited and overcautious in her relationship with the patient. With good reason, she was worried about how her personal problems were going to affect the treatment. Her attitude also became more supportive and sympathetic. Eva and her patient were soon approaching a silent agreement, a collusion, to avoid problems too acute and painful for either of them to deal with.

How should the supervisor behave? How many of her personal problems should they take up within the framework of the supervision?

Cases of supervision

Every participant (trainee supervisor) takes on the regular supervision of a therapist and his psychotherapy. Of course, there are occasions when either the patient breaks off his treatment or the therapist for various reasons cannot fulfil his contract. The trainee supervisor and training supervisor then continue the task with a new patient or therapist, respectively. The supervision concerns itself only with psychodynamic individual therapy. Usually the psychotherapy is carried out with a frequency of one session per week.

Supervising the supervision

An important intermediate aim is integrating theory with practice. As well as processing theoretical knowledge and the experiences and emotional reactions in the seminars, we try to achieve this in the supervising of the participants' own supervision work.

This is carried out in closed supervision groups consisiting of four course participants and a teacher. The groups' meetings are coordinated with the theoretical instruction throughout the training at a frequency of two sessions a week.

The supervision groups discuss a variety of problems, amongst them the following:

- how to establish a working alliance with the supervisee so that the essential dynamic factors in the relationship between patient, therapist, and supervisor can be studied;
- the ways in which the supervisor defines his role as supervisor within an organization;
- the ways in which a supervisor can support and encourage the therapist's own personal style;
- how to encourage and enhance the therapist's ability to work intuitively and independently;
- how the supervisor can assess the therapist's suitability and competence in connection with psychotherapeutic work.

The goals for supervising the supervision are, of course, very similar to psychotherapy supervision. Like the psychotherapy supervisor, the teacher in the supervision group functions as a model in relation to the participants. A great part of the learning of methods and behaviour occurs here, too, in the relation between teacher and trainee supervisor and in the relation to the fellow students in the group. Parallel processes in the chain of patient/therapist/supervisor/teacher may be extremely clear and form a valuable basis for understanding and learning in the supervision group.

Students in the child and adolescent therapeutic training at the Erica Foundation write comprehensive summaries of their therapy cases every year. With a background of the extremely positive experience from writing these summaries, it seemed natural to transfer this element to the supervision training, too. Thus, every participant has an assignment to write a *summary of the supervision process*. For reasons of confidentiality, these are presented only in the supervision group in the presence of a member of the training committee. As with the therapy summaries, these summaries of the supervision have also proved to be of great value. They have often actively contributed to clarification and increasing understanding of the processes that take place during the supervision period between patient–therapist, therapist–supervisor, and supervisor–teacher and the supervision group.

The overall goal for supervision training has been to train competent psychotherapy supervisors and help them develop a professional identity as supervisors. Supervising the supervision has been of greatest importance in this effort.

After the course has been passed the student receives a Certificate in the Supervision and Teaching of Psychotherapy. This certificate is a requirement for a psychotherapist to be a supervisor in the various approved Swedish trainings of psychotherapists that lead to a Government Licence to practice.

REFERENCES

Adelson, M. J. (1995). Clinical supervision of therapists with difficult-to-treat patients. *Bulletin of the Menninger Clinic, 59*: 32–52.

Appelbaum, S. A. (1978). Pathways to change in psychoanalytic psychotherapy. *Bulletin of the Menninger Clinic, 43*: 239–251.

Arlow, J. A. (1963). The supervisory situation. *Journal of the American Psychoanalytic Association, 11 (3)*: 576–594.

Balint, M. (1964). *The Doctor, His Patient and the Illness*. London: Pitman.

Baudry, F. D. (1993). The personal dimension and management of the supervisory situation with a special note on the parallel process. *Psychoanalytic Quarterly, 62*: 588–614.

Bell, D. (1996). Primitive mind of state. *Psychoanalytic Psychotherapy, 10*: 45–58.

Bernard, J. M., & Goodyear, R. K. (1992). *Fundamentals of Clinical Supervision*. Boston: Allyn & Bacon.

Bion, W. R. (1962). *Learning From Experience*. London: Heinemann. [Reprinted London: Karnac Books, 1984.]

Blanck, G., & Blanck, R. (1974). *Ego Psychology: Theory and Practice*. New York: Columbia University Press.

Blomfield, O. H. D. (1985). Psychoanalytic supervision. An overview. *International Review of Psycho-Analysis, 12* (4): 401–410.

Bollas, C. (1992). *Being a Character: Psychoanalysis and Self Experience.* London: Routledge.

Bouchard, M., Normandin, L., & Séguin, M. (1995). Countertransference as instrument and obstacle: A comprehensive and descriptive framework. *Psychoanalytic Quarterly, 44* (4): 717–745.

Bowlby, J. (1980). *Attachment and Loss, Vol. 3.* London: Hogarth Press.

Bromberg, P. (1982). The supervisory process and parallel processes. *Contemporary Psychoanalysis, 18*: 92–94.

Caligor, L. (1984). Parallel and reciprocal processes in psychoanalytic supervision. *Contemporary Psychoanalysis, 17*: 1–27.

Casullo, A., & Resnizky, S. (1993). Supervisión Psicoanalítica: Enfoque Clínico. Reflexiones Clínicas Compartidas. Paper presented at the Sixth Conference on Training Analysis, Amsterdam.

Coderch, J. (1995). *La interpretación en Psicoanálisis. Fundamentos y teoría de la técnica.* Barcelona: Herder.

Corominas, J. (1991). *Psicopatologia i Desenvolupaments Arcaics.* Barcelona: Espaxs.

DeBell, D. E. (1963). A critical digest of the literature on psychoanalytic supervision. *Journal of the American Psychoanalytic Association, 11* (5): 546–575.

Dispaux, M.-F. (1994). How to become a psychotherapist with a psychoanalytic orientation: the place of supervision in the training process. "A good enough training for psychoanalytic psychotherapy: matters of process, identity and psychic change." EFPP Adult Section, European Conference, Luxembourg (October).

Ekstein, R., & Wallerstein, R. (1958). *The Teaching and Learning of Psychotherapy.* New York: Basic Books.

Erikson, E. H. (1963). *Childhood and Society.* New York: W. W. Norton.

Festinger, L. (1957). *A Theory of Cognitive Dissonance.* Stanford, CA: Stanford University Press.

Fleming, J., & Benedek, T. F. (1966). *Psychoanalytic Supervision: A Method of Clinical Teaching.* New York: Grune & Stratton.

Folch, P., & Esteve, J. O. (1992). Multiplicité de la psyché dans les groupes. *Revue de Psychothérapie Psychanalytique de Groupe, 18:* 39–51.

Folch, Terttu Eskelinen de (1981). Some notes on transference and countertransference problems in supervision. *Bulletin of the European Psychoanalytical Federation, 16*: 45–54.

Freud, S. (1912). Recommendations to physicians practicing psychoanalysis. *S.E., 12.*

Freud, S. (1914). Remembering, repeating and working through. *S.E., 12.*

Frijling-Schreuder, E. C. M. (1970). On individual supervision. *International Journal of Psycho-Analysis, 51 (3)*: 363–370.

Fürstenau, P. (1978). *Zur Theorie Psychoanalytischer Praxis.* Stuttgart: Klett-Cotta.

Gabbard, G. O. (1992). The therapeutic relationship in psychiatric hospital treatment. *Bulletin of the Menninger Clinic, 56*: 4–19.

Gabbard, G. O. (1995). Countertransference. The emerging common ground. *International Journal of Psycho-Analysis, 76* (3): 475–485.

Gay, P. (1988). *Freud: A Life for Our Time.* New York: W. W. Norton.

Giovacchini, P. (1990). Countertransference and therapeutic impasses. Unpublished lecture presented to the Madrid Psychoanalytic Association.

Glasser, M. (1992). Problems in the psychoanalysis of certain narcissistic disorders. *International Journal of Psycho-Analysis, 73*: 493–503.

Gordan, K. (1996). *Psychotherapy Supervision in Education, Clinical Practice, and Institutions.* Northvale, NJ: Jason Aronson.

Greenburg, L. S. (1984). Task analysis: the general approach. In: L. N. Rice & L. S. Greenburg (Eds.), *Patterns of Change: Intensive Analysis of Psychotherapy Process.* New York: Guilford Press.

Grinberg, L. (1956). Sobre algunos problemas de técnica psicoanalítica determinados por la identificación y contraidentificación proyectivas. *Revista de Psicoanálisis, 13*: 501–511.

Grinberg, L. (1962). On a specific aspect of countertransference due to the patient's projective identification. *International Journal of Psycho-Analysis, 43*: 436–440.

Grinberg, L. (1963). Psicopatología de la identificación y contraidentificación proyectivas y de la contratransferencia. *Revue de Psicoanálisis,* 2 (2): 112–123.

Grinberg, L. (1970). The problems of supervision in psychoanalytic education. *International Journal of Psycho-Analysis, 51* (3): 371–384.

Grinberg, L. (1979). Countertransference and projective counteridentification. *Contemporary Psychoanalysis, 15*: 226.

Grinberg, L. (1986). *La Supervisión Psicoanalítica. Teoría y Práctica*. Madrid: Tecnipublicaciones, S.A.

Grinberg, L. (1990). Theoretical and clinical aspects of supervision. In: *The Goals of Psychoanalysis* (pp. 289–369). London: Karnac Books.

Gross-Doehrman, M. J. (1976). Parallel processes in supervision and psychotherapy. *Bulletin of the Menninger Clinic, 1*: 9–105.

Haesler, L. (1993). Adequate distance in the relationship between supervisor and supervisee. *International Journal of Psycho-Analysis, 74* (3): 547–556.

Heising, G. (1976). Zur psychodynamik der supervision. *Praxis der Psychotherapie, 21*: 185–191.

Horn, T. (1957). Contribution to the phenomenology of the supervisory process. *American Journal of Psychotherapy, 11*: 769–773.

Ithier, B. (1984). Interviews held with J. McDougall and H. Rosenfield. In: D. Voronovsky (Ed.), *El Control, Cuestión para Psicoanalistas* (pp. 40–53). Buenos Aires: Nueva Visión, 1991.

Jacob, P. (1981). The San Francisco project: the analyst at work. In: R. Wallerstein (Ed.), *Becoming a Psychoanalyst. A Study of Psychoanalytic Supervision*. New York: International Universities Press.

Jacobs, D., David, P., & Meyer, D. J. (1995). *The Supervisory Encounter*. New Haven, CT: Yale University Press.

Johan, M. (1992). Scientific proceedings, panel report: "Enactments in psychoanalysis". *Journal of the American Psychoanalytic Association, 40* (3): 827–841.

Joseph, B. (1988). Projective identification: some clinical aspects. In: J. Sandler (Ed.), *Projection, Identification, Projective Identification*. London: Karnac Books.

Keats, J. (1817). *Letters*, edited by M. B. Forman. London: Oxford University Press, 1952.

Kernberg, O. F. (1973). Psychoanalytic object-relations theory, group processes, and administration: toward an integrative theory of hospital treatment. *The Annual of Psychoanalysis, 1*: 363–388.

Kernberg, O. F. (1984). *Severe Personality Disorders*. New Haven, CT: Yale University Press.

Klein, M. (1935). A contribution to the psychogenesis of manic–depressive states. In: *Love, Guilt and Reparation and Other Works 1921–1945: The Writings of Melanie Klein, Vol. 1*. London: Hogarth Press, 1975. [Reprinted London: Karnac Books, 1992.]

Korn, S., & Carmignani, R. (1987). Process notes as derivative communication about the supervisory field. *Yearbook of Psychoanalysis and Psychotherapy, 2*: 68–84.

Langs, R. (1979). *The Supervisory Experience*. New York: Jason Aronson.

Langs, R. (1992). *A Clinical Workbook for Psychotherapists*. London: Karnac Books.

Langs, R. (1993). *Empowered Psychotherapy*. London: Karnac Books.

Langs, R. (1994). *Doing Supervision and Being Supervised*. London: Karnac Books.

Langs, R. (1995). *Clinical Practice and the Architecture of the Mind*. London: Karnac Books.

Langs, R. (1996). *The Evolution of the Emotion Processing Mind. With an Introduction to Mental Darwinism*. London: Karnac Books.

Langs, R. (1997). *Death Anxiety and Clinical Practice*. London: Karnac Books.

Langs, R. (in press). *Rules, Frames, and Boundaries in Psychotherapy and Counselling*. London: Karnac Books.

Lebovici, S. (1970). Technical remarks on the supervision in psychoanalytic education. *International Journal of Psycho-Analysis, 51*: 385–392.

Loewald, H. (1960). On the therapeutic action of psychoanalysis. *International Journal of Psychoanalysis, 41*: 16–33.

Mackinnon, L. (1986). Supervision and supervision of supervision. *Australian and New Zealand Journal of Family Therapy, 7* (3).

Mackinnon, R. A., Glick, R. A., & Neutzel, E. (1986). Teaching psychoanalytic psychotherapy: The use of the treatment summary. *Journal of Psychiatric Education, 10* (3).

Marcelli, D. (1983). La position Autistique. Hypotèses Psychopathologiques. *Psychiatrie de l'enfant, 26*: 1–16.

Marcus, S. (1985). Freud and Dora: story, history and case story. In: C. Bernheimer & C. Kahane (Eds.), *In Dora's Case* (pp. 56–91). London: Virago Press.

Meltzer, D. (1992). *The Claustrum*. Perth: Clunie Press.

Menzies-Lyth, I. (1960). The functioning of a social system as a defence against anxiety. *Human Relations, 13*: 95–121. [Republished as Tavistock Pamphlet No 3. London: Tavistock Institute of Human Relations, 1970.]

Minnes, P. M. (1987). Ethical issues in supervision. *Canadian Psychology, 28* (3): 285-290.

Ogden, T. (1989). *The Primitive Edge of Experience*. London: Jason Aronson.

Olivier, C. (1995). *Los Hijos de Orestes, o la cuestión del Padre*. Buenos Aires: Nueva Visión.

Piaget, J. (1958). *The Development of Thought: Equilibration of Cognitive Structures*. New York: Viking.

Popper, K. (1972). *Objective Knowledge*. Oxford: Clarendon Press.

Rosenfeld, H. (1971). A clinical approach to the psychoanalytic theory of the life and death instincts: an investigation into the aggressive aspects of narcissism. *International Journal of Psycho-Analysis, 52*: 169–178.

Roughton, R. E. (1993). Useful aspects of acting out: repetition, enactment, and actualization. *Journal of the American Psychoanalytic Association, 41*: 443–472.

Sachs, D. M. (1993). Introductory remarks. Unpublished paper given at the Sixth Conference of IPA Training Analysts, Amsterdam.

Sachs, D. M., & Shapiro, S. H. (1976). On parallel processes in therapy and teaching. *Psychoanalytic Quarterly, 45*: 394–415.

Salvendy, J. T. (1993). Control and power in supervision. *International Journal of Group Psychotherapy, 43*: 363–376.

Sandell, R. (1985). Influence of supervision, therapist's competence and patient's ego level on the effect of timelimited therapy. *Psychotherapy and Psychosomatics, 44*: 103–109.

Sandler, J., & Sandler, A. (1978). On the development of object relationship and affects. *International Journal of Psycho-Analysis, 59*: 285–296.

Schlesinger, H. J. (1981). General principles of psychoanalytic supervision. In: R. Wallerstein (Ed.), *Becoming a Psychoanalyst: A Study of Psychoanalytic Supervision* (pp. 29–38). New York: International Universities Press.

Segal, H. (1981). Countertransference. In: *The Work of Hanna Segal*. New York: Jason Aronson.

Shevrin, H. (1981). Supervision and treatment, as seen from the analyst's perspective. In: R. Wallerstein (Ed.), *Becoming a Psychoanalyst. A Study of Psychoanalytic Supervision* (pp. 227–268). New York: International Universities Press.

Solnit, E. (1970). Learning from psychoanalytic supervision. *International Journal of Psycho-Analysis, 51* (3): 359–362.

Steiner, J. (1993). *Psychic Retreats*. London: Routledge.

Stimmel, B. (1995). Resistance to awareness of the supervisor's transference with special reference to the parallel process. *International Journal of Psycho-Analysis, 76* (6): 609–618.

Styczynski, L. (1980). The transition from supervisee to supervisor. In: A. K. Hess (Ed.), *Psychotherapy Supervision* (pp. 29–40). New York: John Wiley.

Szecsödy, I. (1986). Feedback in psychotherapy and training. *Nordisk Psykiatrisk Tidskrift, 40*: 193–200.

Szecsödy, I. (1990a). *The Learning Process in Psychotherapy Supervision.* Stockholm: Karolinska Institute. [Academic Dissertation Monograph.]

Szecsödy, I. (1990b). The significance and importance of supervision in psychotherapy training. *Psychotherapy and Psychosomatics, 53*: 86–92.

Szecsödy, I. (1990c). Supervision: a didactic or mutative situation. *Psychoanalytic Psychotherapy, 4*: 245–262.

Szecsödy, I. (1994). Supervision—a complex tool for training. *Scandinavian Psychoanalytic Review, 17*: 119–129.

Szecsödy, I., Kächele, H., & Dreyer, K. (1993). Supervision—an intricate tool for psychoanalytic training. *Zeitschrift für Psychoanalytische Theory und Praxis, 84*: 52–70.

Tucker, L., Bauer, S., Wagner, S., Harlem, D., & Sher, I. (1992). Specialized extended hospital treatment for borderline patients. *Bulletin of the Menninger Clinic, 56*: 465–478.

Vachon, M. L. S. (1995). Staff stress in hospice/palliative care: A review. *Palliative Medicine, 9*: 91–113.

Wallerstein, R. (Ed.) (1981). *Becoming a Psychoanalyst. A Study of Psychoanalytic Supervision.* New York: International Universities Press.

Welldon, E. V. (1992). *Mother, Madonna Whore.* London: Guilford.

INDEX

For Product Safety Concerns and Information please contact our EU representative GPSR@taylorandfrancis.com
Taylor & Francis Verlag GmbH, Kaufingerstraße 24, 80331 München, Germany

www.ingramcontent.com/pod-product-compliance
Ingram Content Group UK Ltd.
Pitfield, Milton Keynes, MK11 3LW, UK
UKHW022202190926
475702UK00003B/154
9780367327163